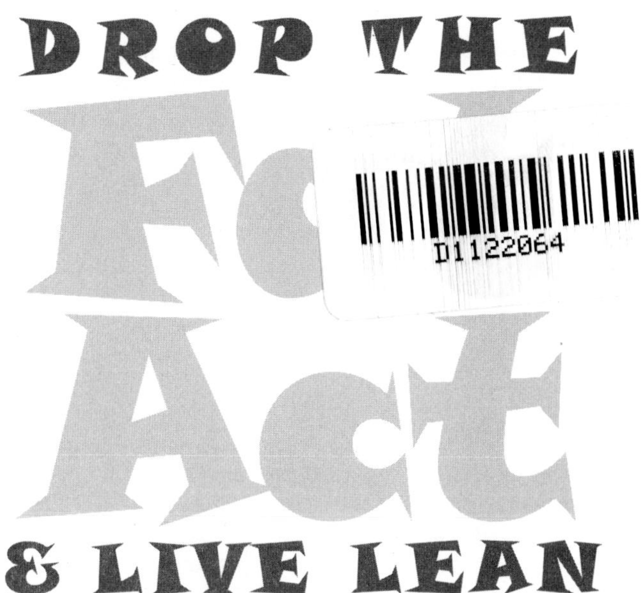

USING THE **OPPOSITES APPROACH** TO **CHANGE YOUR FATTITUDES**

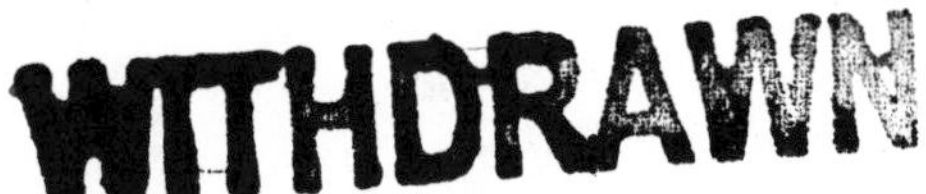

RYAN D. ANDREWS
MS, MA, RD, CSCS

Healthy Living Publications
Summertown, Tennessee

Cover and interior design: Jim Scattaregia
Cover illustration: Brian Farrington

ISBN: 978-1-57067-259-0
Healthy Living Publications
a division of Book Publishing Company
P.O. Box 99
Summertown, TN 38483
888-260-8458
bookpubco.com

Half of the author's proceeds from the sale of this book will be donated to hunger relief efforts and organizations that provide healthful school lunch programs.

Library of Congress Cataloging-in-Publication Data

Andrews, Ryan D.
Drop the fat act and live lean : using the opposites approach to change your fattitudes / Ryan D. Andrews.
p. cm.
Includes bibliographical references and index.
ISBN 978-1-57067-259-0 (pbk.) -- ISBN 978-1-57067-945-2 (e-book)
1. Weight loss--Psychological aspects--Popular works. 2. Food habits--Psychological aspects--Popular works. 3. Exercise--Health aspects--Popular works. 4. Self-care, Health--Popular works. I. Title.
RM222.2.A522 2012
613.2'5--dc23

2011042565

Printed on recycled paper

Book Publishing Company is a member of Green Press Initiative. We chose to print this title on paper with 30% post consumer recycled content, processed without chlorine, which saved the following natural resources:

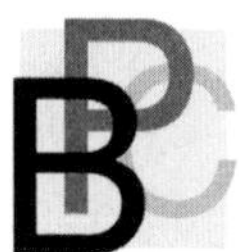

- 10 trees
- 293 pounds of solid waste
- 4,621 gallons of water
- 1,025 pounds of greenhouse gases
- 4 million BTU of energy

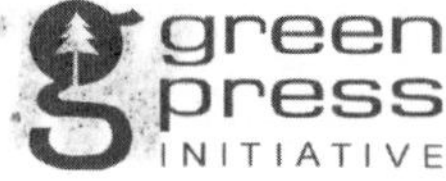

For more information on Green Press Initiative, visit www.greenpressinitiative.org. Environmental impact estimates were made using the Environmental Defense Fund Paper Calculator. For more information visit www.papercalculator.org.

Contents

Foreword

A few years ago I was asked to give a fitness and nutrition seminar in Texas. Now, I love Texas. In fact, I call Texas home for part of the year. However, I have to admit that I was a little intimidated. You see, everything *is* bigger in Texas; including the portion sizes and the people. Indeed, in 2009 Texas had four cities in the list of top ten fattest cities in the United States.

So, faced with the prospect of convincing overly fat, meat-lovin' Texans to clean up their diets and improve their exercise habits, I knew I had to come up with something different. Something other than the old "increase your fiber, eat less saturated fat, and eat more fruits and vegetables" advice.

Sure, eating more fiber, less saturated fat, and more fruits and veggies is important. But everyone already knows that. We've all heard it before. Yet a whopping 97 percent of men and 95 percent of women aren't eating anywhere near the three to five daily servings of fruits and veggies recommended by the American Dietetic Association. Beyond being sad, this is clear evidence that merely telling people to eat more fruits and veggies doesn't work.

But why doesn't it work? For starters, even if you tell people what to eat, and they try to do it, they often fall short. Plus, most people do a pretty lousy job of estimating how their diet stacks up nutritionally. One study showed that participants overestimated the amount of fruits and veggies, as well as lean protein, they were eating, while also underestimating their intake of processed carbohydrates, sugars, and high-fat foods. They thought they were eating more of the good stuff and less of the not-so-good stuff, but they were wrong.

It seems to me that this is the case for most of us—that people tend to overinflate a positive eating decision, such as eating veggies with lunch, while deflating a negative eating decision, such as eating too much ice cream after dinner. Although it's human nature to do this, it can lead to a skewed idea of how you're doing, both personally and in comparison with those around you.

As I geared up for the big Texas event, I knew that my seminar had to help people find a way to short-circuit this behavior pattern. Instead of once again telling the audience to eat more fruits and veggies, I had to do something with greater impact. So I decided to use a little trick called "teaching the opposite."

Instead of giving my Texas audience threadbare rules for being leaner, fitter, and healthier, I decided to give them rules for the opposite outcome. I taught them exactly what they should do to gain body fat, lose muscle, guarantee diabetes and heart disease, and live a shorter life.

The response was incredible. Lightbulbs were going off all over the room. The attendees were seeing something clearly for the first time. Not only did my approach help them realize their habits weren't so good, it also helped them realize that they were regularly engaging in behaviors guaranteed to destroy their bodies, degrade their health, and, ultimately, shorten their lives.

That novel approach is also the key to the effectiveness of the book you're holding in your hands. In *Drop the Fat Act & Live Lean*, my good friend (and master coach) Ryan Andrews clearly outlines the lifestyle, dietary choices, and exercise habits that will assuredly lead to more body fat, less muscle, lifestyle-related disease, poor quality of life, and a shorter life span.

It's all here: how to use breakfast, lunch, and dinner to gain body fat; how to drink your way to diabetes (no alcohol required); how to lose muscle mass, bone mass, and mobility by avoiding exercise; how to use food to manage your feelings and guarantee binge eating; and how saying "I'll start my program on Monday" can actually mean, "I'll never start my program."

"But," you say, "I want the opposite outcomes! I want to be leaner, fitter, and healthier and live longer." That's covered too, but before you can really understand how to live in a way that's consistent with a lean lifestyle, you need to study the opposite: the habits of folks who aren't lean and fit. Only then can you truly understand how to do the opposite.

I know this approach is a little unconventional. However, your new coach, Ryan Andrews, is a somewhat unconventional guy. He's not only an accomplished academic, with two master's degrees and nearly every fitness and nutrition accreditation available, he's also a guy who wears his fitness on his sleeve. From 1996 to 2001 he was a nationally ranked competitive bodybuilder, and he continues to maintain a lean, superfit body while following a plant-based diet that's friendly to both the environment and the physique.

But beyond his street cred and "book cred," Ryan also knows how to coach. He's worked at the Weight Management Center at Johns Hopkins Medicine, one of the most recognized and awarded institutions in the world. He's also heavily involved in the world's largest body transformation project: Precision Nutrition's Lean Eating Coaching Program.

I've often said that the perfect coach is someone with theoretical knowledge, personal experience, and a history of success in helping others. That describes Ryan to a T. So rest assured that you're in good hands. All that's left to do is open your mind and dig in to *Drop the Fat Act & Live Lean*. If you take the lessons in this book to heart—and then do the opposite—a lifetime of leanness awaits.

In health and fitness,

John Berardi, PhD, CSCS
President, Precision Nutrition, Inc.

Editor's Note: *John Berardi is one of North America's most popular and respected authorities on fitness and nutrition. He has made his mark as a leading researcher in the field of exercise and nutritional science, as an author, and as a coach and trainer to thousands of elite athletes and recreational exercisers. You can find out more at precisionnutrition.com.*

Preface

When disturbed by negative thinking, think the opposite.

—Yoga Sutra II:33

We humans are always evolving, aren't we? This seems to be especially true of our values and choices related to eating. One minute we're disciplined, and the next we're reckless. We're confident about our food choices one day, and completely disoriented the next.

No matter where you currently stand in your journey with nutrition, remember that having a lean body isn't about showing off in tight clothes or feeling superior at the next class reunion. That's not it at all. A lean body gives you the opportunity to live a healthful, fulfilling, productive, and purposeful life—a life that betters the planet and those who reside on it.

You might wonder if that claim is a little far-reaching. Look at it this way: How we look influences how we feel. How we feel influences how we live. And how we live influences the world.

While you'll definitely find humor, sarcasm, off-the-wall comments, and some strange analogies in this book, I want to assure you that I don't take health, fitness, and excess body fat lightly. I understand fitness (and fatness) challenges because I've studied them, coached people who face these challenges, and worked through them myself.

When you're lean and healthy, you have the opportunity to live a meaningful life that can make others' lives better. This is the reason my goal is to help people look and feel their best. I hope this book contributes to your journey of becoming the person you dream of being.

Acknowledgments

Thanks to Mom for everything; Dad for challenging me; Dave Hansow for making me a better person; John Berardi, PhD, CSCS, for making me think; Victoria Moran for getting me through life; Shannon Bishop, RD, for giving me a chance; the *Daily Kent Stater* newspaper for allowing me to write; Barbra and Michael Stricker for keeping me real; Steve Riechman, PhD, MPH, for guiding me; Jamie Erskine, PhD, RD, for inspiring me; Johns Hopkins Medicine, Carmen Roberts, MS, RD, and Larry Cheskin, MD, for giving me a life-changing opportunity; Denise Supik, MS, LCPC, for teaching me how to listen and counsel; Jim Rome for positive energy; Steve Nickerson for a new spin on life; Dan "Bizarro" Piraro for the best cartoons ever; Colleen Patrick-Goudreau for giving me hope; the Precision Nutrition team for keeping the science fresh; and Book Publishing Company for making this book happen.

Introduction
Fat Is What Fat Does

For the first time ever, overweight people outnumber average people in America. Doesn't that make overweight the average then? Last month you were fat, now you're average—hey, let's get a pizza!

—Jay Leno

I have bad news: if you live, eat, and exercise like most North Americans, you're fat. How do you know if you're fat? The eyeball test. That isn't something I made up in a frat-house basement with my buddies. I learned about the eyeball test from a medical textbook called *The Merck Manual*. Section 1, chapter 5, of this prestigious medical text reads, "For practical purposes, the eyeball test is sufficient: If a person looks fat, the person is fat."[1] The authors suggest that health practitioners need not bother with technical measurements; we can simply use the eyeball test. I challenge you to do the test, here and now.

If you're fat, you're probably going to die of a preventable disease. Translation: You're probably going to die because of the choices you make each day. What do you think of that? You might think I'm going to try to sell you a magical weight-loss powder to sprinkle on your feet before bed. Sorry, you won't score any magical weight-loss powders from me.

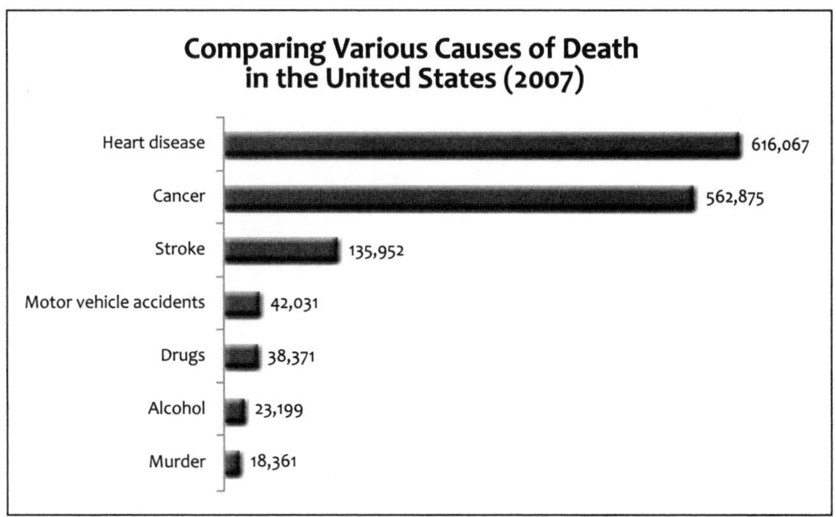

Data from Centers for Disease Control, FastStats (cdc.gov/nchs/fastats/lcod.htm).

Or maybe you have a smirk on your face because you think you're Mr. or Ms. Picture of Health and believe you're way beyond all those unfit losers when it comes to eating and exercise. Perhaps you remove the skin from your boiled chicken thighs and use skim milk on your boxed breakfast cereal. Sorry to wake you up with the bad news, but it's the twenty-first century. If you think skinless chicken, processed grains, and nonfat cow's milk will benefit your health, you're still copping a fattitude.

Habits of the Fat and Unhealthy

I once worked with an obese woman who looked me in the eye and said, with complete seriousness, that she avoided bananas because they're high in calories. She'd heard this from a friend and assumed that bananas would therefore make her fat(ter). (Side note: I'm guessing her friend was fat too.) Meanwhile, for dinner the previous night this client consumed a 16-ounce steak and a deep-fried onion appetizer from a local steakhouse. That's about 2,500 calories in one meal!

Get this: To consume 2,500 calories from bananas, you'd need to eat about twenty-three of them. That's about 6 pounds of bananas! Good luck with that. Better start peeling and chewing. Have you ever eaten just two or three bananas in a row? Holy fullness! The fact is, twenty-three bananas contain about 70 grams of fiber.

Hopefully you're at least one step ahead of that client and recognize that overconsumption of raw fruit isn't a major nutritional concern among the overweight, and that eating raw fruit in place of doughnuts and taquitos would—gasp!—probably improve people's health. Banana benders? I don't see that happening.

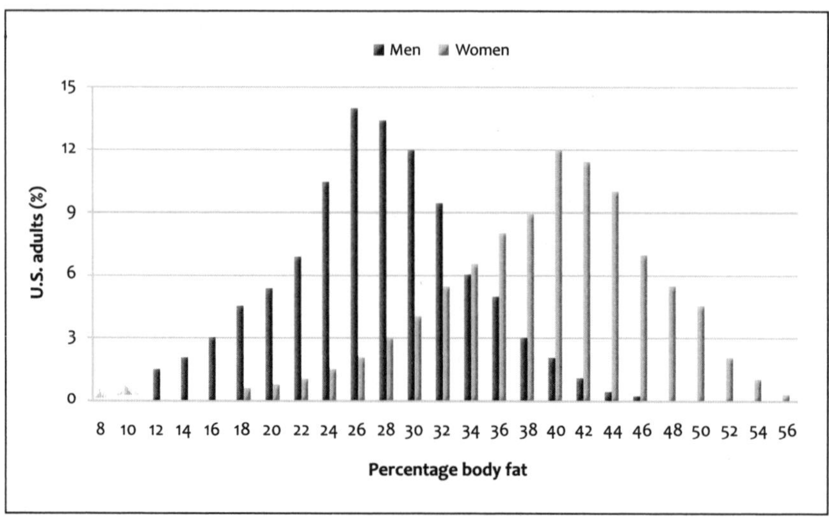

Adapted with permission from *American Journal of Clinical Nutrition* (2009; 90; 1457–1465), American Society for Nutrition.

Sadly, stories like this are not the exception. Fat and the attitudes that promote it are the new "normal," as the graph on the previous page from the *American Journal of Clinical Nutrition* abundantly illustrates.[2]

Nutrition expert Brad Pilon noticed a few remarkable things after reviewing this graph:[3]

- The percentage of body fat seems to be normally distributed across the North American population.
- A man's average body fat is around 25 percent.
- A woman's average body fat is around 40 percent.

These "norms" are unfortunate. For context, the healthy range for percentage of body fat for men is 8 to 25 percent and for women is 21 to 36 percent, depending on age—and you should be aware that the age range extends up to seventy-nine years! The take-away message? If you want to be lean and healthy, you'd best be abnormal. Remember, norms are socially constructed, meaning they're created and maintained by people. The current norm in North America is fat and unhealthy. It's time to look at what most people are doing and start doing things differently.

Fat people have typical habits, beliefs, and personalities that play a role in their fatness. When I'm working with clients who are overweight and trying to figure out why in the heck they've been diagnosed with diabetes, I can practically predict their typical day. I can make a pretty good guess as to how they eat, how they sleep, how they exercise, who they hang out with, and how they've tried to deal with their weight in the past. I've developed this ability through interactions with thousands of clients, dialogues with hundreds of colleagues, data from thousands of books and articles, and general observations of people's behavioral patterns, not to mention spying on family and friends.

The good news is, if you don't follow in the footsteps of fat and unhealthy people, you won't be fat and unhealthy. It would be darn near impossible. If you live like a healthy person, you'll almost assuredly be a healthy person. This is just one of the laws of nature.

Each chapter in parts I through III of this book will cover a habit, behavior, routine, or attitude typical of fat people. If you want to get fat and unhealthy, then, by all means, follow their lead. Do exactly what they do. Heck, you could just move in with a fat person for a few months. Chances are, you'll get fat. But if you want to be lean and healthy and feel great, then walk, or run—or both—in the opposite direction.

You may be thinking I'm a little smug—that I believe my ideas are always 100 percent right on. So let me say up front that I know exceptions are inevitable. So please don't email me saying, "I do [insert bad habit here], but I'm still in decent shape and good health." That's fine. Keep doing what works for you if you want to. But I'll be honest, in the long term the odds aren't in your favor. The ideas presented in this book aren't just theories, and they aren't unique to me. They're built on years of personal observations, not to mention countless research articles.

I know my writing style may not appeal to everybody. I ask that you stick with the book through at least two chapters. If you're still not on board after two chapters, stick with me for one more. At that point, if you're still not down with my ideas (no matter what you think of my writing style), you're just plain wrong. Sorry.

Habits of the Lean and Fit

When I started graduate school, I asked my advisor, Steve Riechman, a simple question: What behaviors do successful graduate students display? He responded with four points:

1. They sit in the front of the classroom.
2. They volunteer to help with research in the department.
3. They volunteer to go first with presentations and projects.
4. They turn in papers before the deadline.

That all made sense to me, so I decided to cultivate those behaviors. Two years and six hundred cups of green tea later, I finished two master's degrees—one in exercise physiology and the other in nutrition. Throughout that time I slept seven to nine hours per night, exercised at least five hours per week, worked part-time as a graduate assistant, worked part-time as a writer for the campus newspaper, and volunteered on Saturday mornings at a food bank—and freely admit that I just couldn't seem to make time for boozing at parties.

Okay, enough reminiscing. Here's my point: During grad school, I did what successful graduate students did. As a result, I was successful. That experiment helped me realize what a powerful strategy mimicry can be, including in the realms of health and weight.

So, are you mimicking the behaviors of those who eat healthful foods, exercise regularly, and successfully lead a fit life? If you are, then you're almost assuredly fit—and you're reading this book because you enjoy my writing. That's fine by me. Then there's the flip side: If you aren't mimicking the success patterns of fit people, you're probably fat and unhealthy.

This idea doesn't click for some people at first—especially regarding themselves. It's usually easier to see how the behavior of others is inconsistent with their priorities. Maybe you know someone who wants to be wealthy but spends a lot of money on scratch cards and then complains about doing entry-level work. Maybe you know people who say they want to spend more time with their kids but can't seem to get off the merry-go-round of workaholism and make time for the playground. Or maybe you know someone who gorges on dessert each night but complains about having a spare tire. (Oops! Maybe that's actually you.) This is a pattern sometimes called the integrity gap.

Right now, take a few moments to consider the habits and character of people who are lean and healthy. Get into the mind-set of people who are lean and healthy, then answer the following questions:

- What do they eat for breakfast? For lunch? For dinner?
- How often do they exercise and what kinds of exercise do they do?
- Do they enjoy exercising and eating nutritious food?
- Who are their friends?
- Are they optimists or pessimists? Assertive or passive? Happy or unhappy?
- How do they feel when they look in the mirror?

Next, answer these same questions from the mind-set of people who are fat and unhealthy. Does this give you any insight into how a fat, unhealthy person lives and views the world?

Now for the really hard part: How do your own daily habits stack up in comparison? Do you do any of the following on a regular basis?

- Skip breakfast and make dinner your largest meal
- Eat quickly, haphazardly, and while doing other things
- Count calories and go on diets
- Regularly eat processed foods and refined grains
- Drink high-calorie beverages
- Eat out frequently
- Exercise fewer than four hours per week
- Get inadequate sleep
- Use food to manage your feelings
- Watch two or more hours of television per day
- Hang out with fat people

Beyond Self-Image and Self-Interest

You may not have much concern about the average overweight consumer indulging in a 12-ounce steak each Saturday night, but I do—and not just because it's a recipe for clogged arteries, colon polyps, and unpleasant body odor. I also care because I don't want to run out of fresh water. Producing 1 pound of beef can use up to 1,800 gallons of water (depending on the production methods).[4] Folks, a six-minute shower uses 15 gallons, and that's a pretty long shower. Think of it like this: if you didn't shower for four months, you'd conserve only about 1,800 gallons of water—the same quantity of water required to produce a single pound of beef.

You may be thinking, "But, Ryan, I only buy beef that's [grass-fed, organic, humane, locally grown—whatever]." Good. That's a step in the right direction. There are ways to produce beef that are more sustainable. But you know what's *really* sustainable? Plants. In the United States, 157 million tons of protein from grains, legumes, and vegetables are fed to livestock to yield just 28 million tons of protein in the form of meat.[5] Plus, eating plant protein doesn't require any rationalizations. If we find ourselves in our species' final hours on this planet, surrounded by sewage-laden water and toxic air and soil, and you have 20 pounds of beef in your basement freezer, I'd hate to have to say I told you so—not a very pleasant fare-thee-well.

Then there's the human equation. Our planet currently has about the same number of overweight individuals as it does hungry and malnourished people: nearly one billion.[6] Why the disparity? A big part of it is the statistics I just mentioned, regarding how much of the food produced each day in the United States is used as animal feed, and this isn't because we're overburdened with pet hamsters. This food is fed to livestock to satisfy Americans' ever-increasing demand for meat. The Worldwatch Institute summed it up well: "In 1990, . . . the World Hunger Program at Brown University calculated that recent world harvests, if

Eat plenty of fruit & learn to multiply. That way you won't pollute your bodies & the earth with animal agriculture, & reproduce faster than the planet can support.
We should have written that down. What was it again?
"Be fruitful & multiply," I think.
BIZARRO.COM
PIRARO 3-19-08

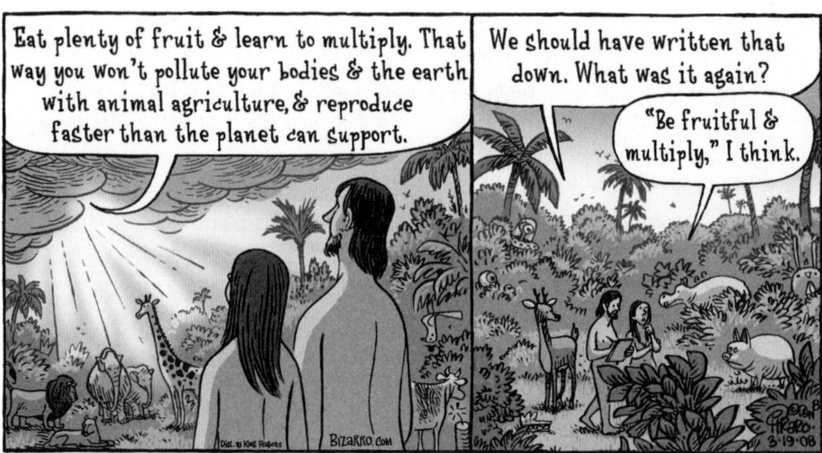

Bizarro, reprinted by permission of Dan Piraro.

equitably distributed with no diversion of grain to feeding livestock, could provide a vegetarian diet to 6 billion people, whereas a meat-rich diet like that of people in the wealthier nations could support only 2.6 billion."[7]

The average American adult eats about 222 pounds of meat per year, a figure that doesn't include seafood.[8] And how many Americans eat a plant-based diet? Diddly-point-squat. In the United States, there are more people who believe we've made contact with aliens than who eat a completely plant-based diet.[9–11] When it comes to marine life, you're probably well aware of the current craze for eating seafood rich in omega-3 fatty acids. Regardless of the nutritional benefits, this is putting more pressure on an already strained resource. If overfishing and marine pollution continue, we may see a complete collapse of the world's fish populations by the year 2048.[12]

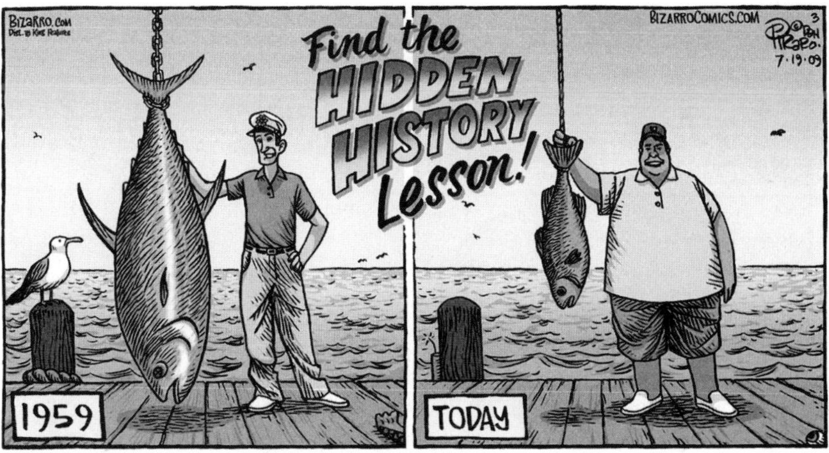

Bizarro, reprinted by permission of Dan Piraro.

Beyond feeding a lot of food to farm animals, Americans feed a lot of food to trash cans. In the United States, 20 to 25 percent of all food purchased for the home is wasted. If that doesn't seem galling, try this experiment: Go to the grocery store and buy five bags of groceries. Then take one bag directly to a dumpster and throw it in. Americans do this so regularly that the waste adds up to about 474.5 pounds of food per year.[13, 14]

Are you sick of hearing about these issues yet? I am. So why am I bringing them up? For incentive. Sure, you might sit down to a plant-based meal in the hopes of lowering your cholesterol or looking better in a tank top. But those types of reasons seem kind of lame in comparison to the big picture. If you're motivated to alter your food choices because of concerns about world hunger, fresh water supplies, environmental sustainability, and animal welfare, holy cow! That's almost seven billion people and billions more animals rooting for you to make the right decision. Don't let them all down.

Incentives

Bob Harper called and he wants his legumes back. You know who Bob is, right? The tough trainer who has kicked people into shape on the hit reality show *The Biggest Loser*? I think you'd agree that he seems like a gnarly dude. Did you know that he eats an entirely plant-based diet? In case you hadn't guessed it yet, so do I. Many folks think a plant-based (aka vegan) diet makes people scrawny. In a way, I agree. Most vegans I meet are thin. Yet I find it fascinating that scrawny vegetarians are so often frowned upon, especially in the United States, a nation where 70 percent of the population is far too fat and about $140 billion per year is devoted to treating obesity-related diseases.[15]

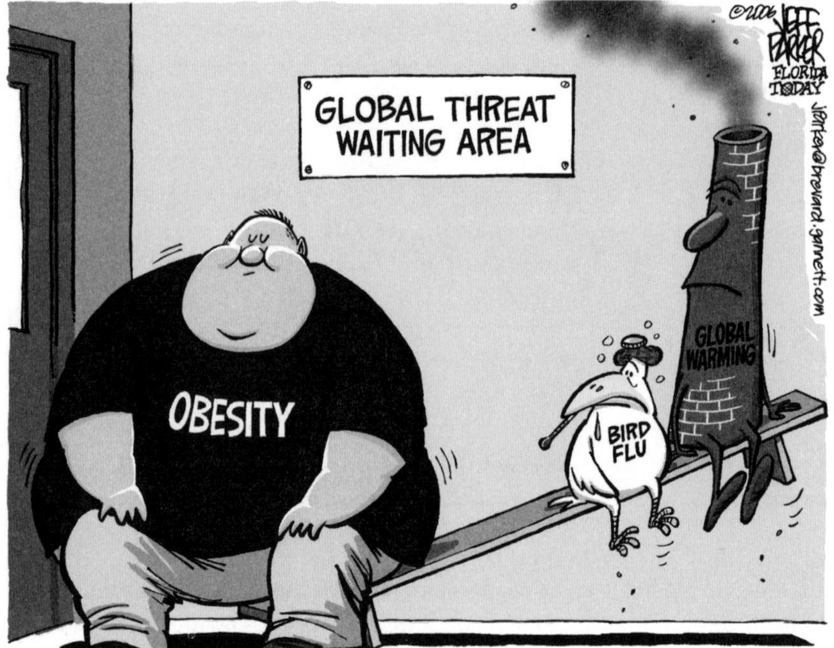

Reprinted by permission of caglecartoons.com.

After working with many vegans—and having eaten a plant-based diet myself for several years—I feel like I finally have a good perspective on why vegans tend to be thin, and it has to do with incentives. Many vegans are lean for a few key reasons:

- They want to use fewer resources and create less waste.
- They want to spend less money on food.
- They feel full and satisfied after eating a whole-foods, plant-based, high-fiber meal.
- They enjoy being strong and healthy and walk or bike or take the stairs whenever they can.

Compelling Motivations

Between the ages of fourteen and twenty I was a competitive bodybuilder, and my concerns about diet revolved around how it influenced my body and performance. My main considerations about any given food were whether it would lower my body fat and increase my muscle mass and whether it would improve my chances of winning a contest.

After I hung up my posing trunks, my motivations around diet evolved. I started thinking about how my eating habits influenced my long-term health and asking questions like "Will it increase my chances of developing heart disease and cancer?" These days I have yet another set of considerations about food:

- Is it harmful to animals, other people, or the environment?
- Does it support my physical, emotional, and spiritual health?
- Does it support farmers and human rights?
- Why the hell am I thinking about so many issues before I eat?

Looking back on my own journey, I wonder whether people who have difficulty eating a nutritious diet simply don't have compelling incentives. How many people stick with a healthful diet for the rest of their lives for the following reasons?

- They want to look fit for an upcoming class reunion.
- They want to lower their cholesterol because their doctor scared them.
- They want to look buff on the beach in Mexico.
- They read in a magazine that carbs are bad.

I'm guessing not many. If you really want to make a lifelong change, your incentives for eating differently need to be meaningful. Although eating for the sole purpose of looking lean and muscular was a very powerful motivator for me at one point in time, it simply isn't compelling enough on its own to support an enduring change.

Developing a New Social Norm

Here's what it comes down to: Lean people don't get that way by "dieting"; they live lean lives. They eat the right amount of nutritious food for optimal health and vitality, and they exercise their bodies on a regular basis. They're motivated to live this way because it's meaningful to them and integrated with a higher sense of purpose.

What if this way of living were the social norm? We human beings tend to take our social norms seriously: we help our friends move, we hold the door open for others, and we volunteer our time for charitable causes—and we do these things willingly, not because we expect immediate payback, or necessarily any payback at all. Having similar norms for healthful eating and living a lean lifestyle could provide powerful motivation and meaningful incentives.

Results and Not Excuses

Did you know that people still smoke? Seriously. About 21 percent of Americans smoke,[16] even though they're well aware of the probability of developing a disease—quite possibly a fatal disease—as a result. Knowing this, do I still have hope that a majority of North Americans will adopt a lifestyle of eating healthful plant-based foods and exercising on a regular basis? Ha! Not in my lifetime.

Most people prefer to live in a dietary La-La Land, telling themselves that what they eat won't end up killing them. Sure, sometimes they suffer through exercise and eating collard greens, rice, and black beans, but only because they have their eye on the "prize": maybe a cigarette, a double margarita, a triple-bacon-cheeseburger, or deep-fried butter balls (I kid you not). But are unhealthful behaviors actually a reward? Do they genuinely enrich people's lives? Or do people perhaps indulge in these death-inducing habits simply because that's the social norm?

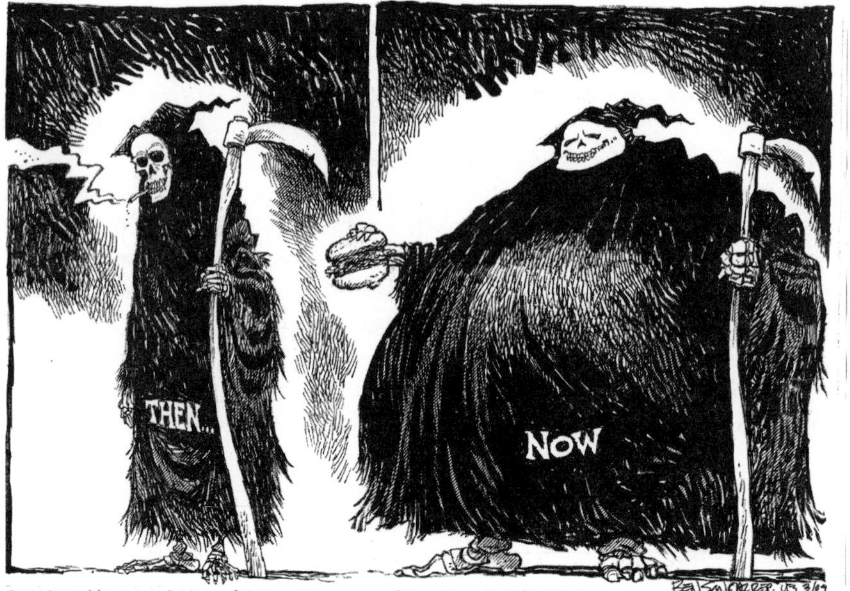

Reprinted by permission of Steve Benson and Creators Syndicate, Inc.

Values versus Preferences

Once people are finally armed with all of the information necessary to make positive changes to their diets and lifestyles, they often still have to overcome a huge hurdle: the excuse "But I like my ______."

If I'm talking about plant-based eating, people say, "But I like my meat." If I'm talking about bringing lunch from home, people say, "But I like my fast food." If I'm talking about drinking green tea, people say, "But I like my soda." If I'm talking about lifting weights, people say, "But I like my beanbag chair at home."

These are understandable rationales—if you're still in kindergarten. Kids may say they like taunting siblings, eating dessert before dinner, or yelling at the top of their lungs while you're on the phone. But liking something doesn't necessarily validate doing it or make it a good idea. Heck, I like cigars and ice cream, but I don't indulge in them. Why? I know it's a bad idea, even if I think I like them.

These examples may seem obvious. But is it really any different if you use this excuse to allow yourself to eat crappy food, skip a workout, or engage in another unhealthful activity? By the way, don't get too fixated on the word "like"; you may phrase it differently. You might justify your behavior by saying, "I need a break," "I'm not perfect," or, my favorite, "Everything in moderation." How lame is that?

The truth is, the immediate satisfaction we obtain from something is a powerful motivator. Yet as we get older and wiser, we begin to realize that choices that feel difficult or unpleasant in the moment often have consequences that we like in the long run. So you might choose to do something that isn't very fun right now because you like the long-term results.

A successful CEO may not always like taking on extra projects, but she chooses to do so because she values running the company and providing a reliable product or service. Someone on a plant-based diet might not always like eating a healthful home-cooked meal instead of going out for steak, but he may choose to do so anyway knowing that his dinner choice didn't come at the cost of an animal's life—or a triple bypass on down the road. A volunteer may not always like showing up at the animal shelter with a smile on her face, but she chooses to do so because she feels good about helping solve the problem of pet overpopulation in the community. A stay-at-home father may not always like cleaning up after the kids, doing laundry, and preparing meals, but he chooses to do so because he feels it's important to instill his values in his kids. An athlete might not always like going to practice instead of watching TV, but she chooses to do so anyway because she wants to improve her skills, and her chances of winning. And the list goes on.

Successful people don't always like what they're doing in the moment, but they choose to do it anyway because they value the long-term outcome. Liking something in the moment isn't a requirement for success. The only requirement is that the behavior gets you closer to your goals and what you care about in life. This is good news, right? You can like the healthful option because it aligns with your vision for the future. With time, you may begin to like the process because it's aligned with your core values.

Choosing How You Want to Live

People contact me asking for advice about nutrition and exercise. They get excited and want to live a fit life. But all too often they conjure up an array of excuses as to why the time isn't right to change their habits. At this point, they often look at me expectantly, hoping I can provide the psychological equivalent of a magical weight-loss powder—some sort of hocus-pocus motivation that will help them succeed. After they discover I don't have a magic wand that will make them commit to lifestyle changes, many of them decide they don't have it within themselves to change their ways. The truth? It isn't that they are unable to change; rather, it comes down to whether (or how much) they actually *want* to change.

A 2010 survey revealed that three out of four Americans would give up their television, cell phones, and computers to get lean.[17] But wait—then why are so many people texting friends and watching *Man v. Food* marathons all weekend? The survey also indicated that more Americans would rather lose weight than get promoted at work. But wait—then why are so many Americans working ten-hour days? Cognitive dissonance alert! What these people are actually doing is deluding themselves. They don't really want to eat healthfully and exercise; it's just a fleeting notion that excites them. If they were actually ready to make a change, they'd do it without rationalizing why they can't. Here's one final statistic from that survey to shed some light on the sad truth about why 46 percent of Americans decided not to change their eating habits, even if they thought they needed to lose weight: They didn't want to give up certain foods. Yep, it boiled down to "But I like my _____."

People who are ready to make a change simply make the change. I'll share something about myself that may be relevant here: I've come to realize that whenever I'm feeling kind of depressed (which, fortunately, isn't often), it's because I'm ignoring the fact that I need to make a change in my life. There is something I need to face, and failing to do so is depressing. Sound familiar?

Actions Speak Louder Than Words

Take a look at your schedule. It doesn't lie. It tells you what you care about. The following passage from Robin Sharma's book *The Greatness Guide* expresses this perfectly:

> There's an old phrase that says "what you're doing speaks so loudly I cannot hear what you are saying." You can say that your primary value involves putting your family first, but if time with your family is not all over your schedule, well then the *truth* of the matter is that your family life isn't your priority. You can say that being in world-class physical condition is another top value but if I don't see five or six workouts etched into your weekly schedule, then the reality to be confronted is that your health just isn't as important as you profess it to be. You can argue that self-development is an essential pursuit to you because the better you are, the more effective you'll be. Show me your schedule and I'll discover the truth. Because your schedule doesn't lie.
>
> There can be no authentic success and lasting happiness if your daily schedule is misaligned with your deepest values. That's a big idea that has been so helpful to so many of the executive clients that I coach. If there is a gap between what you do and who you are, you are out of integrity. I call it the integrity gap. . . . You are not walking your talk. . . .
>
> Your schedule is the best barometer for what you truly value and believe to be important. Too many people talk a good talk. But talk is cheap. Show me your schedule and I'll show you what your priorities are.[18]

Feeling Upset?

You might be feeling a little upset right now. You might feel threatened by my insinuations—hell, my accusations—that you are responsible if you're fat. Maybe you feel like your back is against the wall. That's great! Because that's when we make dramatic changes.

People generally prefer to stay in their comfort zone, fine-tuning their reasons for dodging change. Why would you want to change if what you're doing feels comfortable and, dare I say, effortless. Why would you want to give that up? Just remember, whatever you're doing in life right now is exactly what you want to be doing. Making a change is up to you. But the least I can do is lend you a hand. That's why I hope I've taken you out of your comfort zone.

At this point, I bet you think I'm a hard-ass. You're right! I didn't get to be a successful coach by encouraging people to take the easy way out. But I also know that we're all unique. So just because I suggest something in this book, that doesn't mean you absolutely must do it. Although all of my recommendations will be useful and effective for most people, don't forget to apply common sense and focus on the approaches that work for you.

Section I:
The Fat Eater

Chapter 1
Fat People Skip Breakfast and Make Dinner Their Largest Meal

Eat breakfast like a king, lunch like a prince, and dinner like a pauper.

—Adelle Davis

These days, skipping breakfast and eating a huge dinner seems to be almost as American as baseball.[1–4] (So maybe we shouldn't be too surprised that folks often still seem to make room for half of that iconic apple pie.) Unfortunately, if you skip breakfast, your chances of getting (or being) fat *quadruple*.[2] What's the answer? I hate to break it to you, but it isn't hitting up the local breakfast buffet. In my view, one of the top contenders for worst nutrition cliché has got to be "Always eat breakfast." It's totally lame because it doesn't give any guidance on what to eat. Those who actually take that nugget of advice too often see it as carte blanche to gorge on doughnuts, sausage biscuits, and tubes of yogurt.

What's that you say? Doughnuts, sausage biscuits, and tubes of yogurt are all you have time to eat in the morning? You're not alone. In the United States, the average adult spends only thirty-two minutes each day on food prep and cleanup. Assuming that a full one-third of that time is devoted to breakfast (which seems a bit unlikely), that means most people dedicate only ten minutes or so to breakfast. Even worse, the average male college student devotes less than seven minutes to the first meal of the day. Oh well, I guess that's to be expected. I mean, they did have a long, rigorous night of beer drinking, throwing things down the dorm trash chute, and Xbox tournaments.

Personally, I think good nutrition is worth devoting some time to. But no matter where you stand on that point, limited time just doesn't cut it as an excuse. There are plenty of nutritious breakfast options that you can make in ten minutes—or seven for that matter. You can eat leftovers, which require no prep whatsoever. Or you can blend fruit, nondairy milk, and perhaps some leafy greens to make a breakfast shake. And don't overlook the tried-but-true option of a bowl of oatmeal or whole-grain granola with nondairy milk—it may seem mundane, but at least one study shows that those who eat this kind of breakfast tend to have a lower body mass index than those who skip the morning meal.[3]

Although nearly 90 percent of Americans acknowledge that breakfast is a good idea, about 30 percent don't eat it.[1–4] For those eating breakfast, what are they choosing? When I last checked, sales for the fast-food breakfast market were about $55 billion, so I'm guessing that most people aren't choosing healthful stuff.[5]

When people eat breakfast at home, the most popular items include ready-to-eat cereals, milk, and coffee. When people eat breakfast away from home, the most popular items include bacon, bagels, coffee, eggs, pastries, and sausage. The people in North America who most often skip breakfast include those between the ages of twelve and twenty-nine, African Americans, and low-income families.[1–4, 6]

Riding a Vicious Cycle

Now, I'm not an idiot. And even if I'm treating *you* like one, I know you're not either. I realize that most people understand that eating a nutritious breakfast is a good idea. There are two main reasons fat people skip breakfast: First, they're still full from eating a supersized dinner the previous night. And second, their guilt about eating so much food the night before makes them think that forgoing breakfast—and maybe lunch—is a good way to cut calories. Unfortunately, when dinnertime rolls around they're ravenous after another day of not eating, so they binge and the cycle begins again.

Sadly, eating a huge dinner is often just the beginning of strapping on the evening feedbag. If I had a nickel for every client who admitted to continuing to snack after dinner to the point of feeling bloated, I'd have at least $13.15. Needless to say, it happens a lot. Night eaters consume at least 25 percent of their total daily calories after dinner.[7] And let's be real. People aren't parking on the couch in front of the TV with a big bowl of romaine. This also circles back to the aforementioned guilt

... and though science has not found that watching TV causes obesity, we do know that stuffing your face, with or without the TV on, does. Back to you, Dave.
HEALTH NEWS
Streeter
Reprinted by permission of cartoonstock.com.

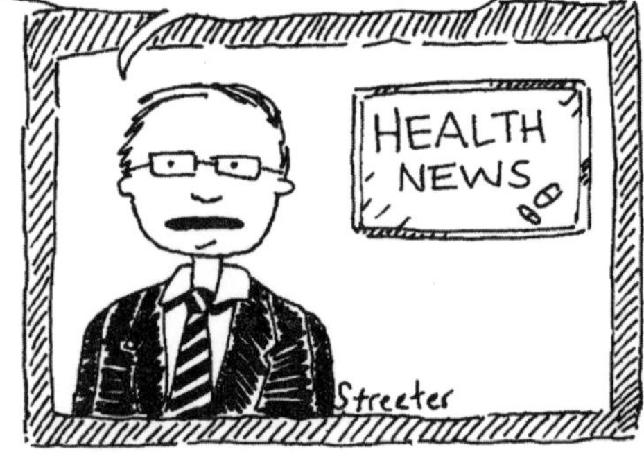

factor. Overeating at night leaves people feeling like they blew it. So they wake up, skip breakfast, and continue to ride the vicious cycle (which, I might add, is an exercise in futility).

Once upon a time I was working with a 275-pound man who regularly ate yogurt for breakfast. He had heard on TV that it was a good idea to eat a container of yogurt for breakfast. (News flash: Getting advice on health and nutrition from TV commercials is a bad idea.) Meanwhile, he skipped lunch and then made a nightly pizza run—and I'm not talking two slices of veggie pizza. He was regularly ordering a large, cheesy, meaty, death-inducing pizza and eating the entire thing.

He couldn't understand why he was ravenous when dinner rolled around. Hmm, could it maybe be because he was expecting a small container of artificially sweetened cultured cattle juice to keep him nourished for a majority of the day? Eventually, I talked this client into switching to a bowl of oatmeal with berries and hempseeds (the latter for protein and omega-3 fatty acids) instead. His pizza benders eventually became a thing of the past and the pounds started dropping.

Let's be real. If you don't eat quality food in the morning, you're setting yourself up for intense feelings of hunger later in the day. And here's the bad news: the cravings you get probably won't be for lentils or roasted beets, if for no other reason than that these aren't convenience foods. Chances are you'll satisfy those hunger pangs with whatever you can find at the corner store.

Making Sure You Feel Like Gorging

The fact is, your body does a much better job of managing hunger, supplying sustained energy, and digesting food when you eat smaller meals at shorter, even intervals. So if you want to be fat and unhealthy, be sure to eat huge amounts of food in one sitting.

If you don't believe me, consider this: Researchers at the University of Massachusetts found that men who don't eat in the morning are almost five times more likely to be obese than those who make breakfast an everyday habit.[8] Likewise, a study of over 2,200 adolescents found that the more regularly the kids ate something for breakfast, the leaner they were. Those who skipped meal numero uno were fatter.[9] The implication is obvious: eat reasonable meals throughout the day. This is easier to do if you wake up hungry and ready to eat. Translation: Don't hit up a buffet twenty minutes before bedtime.

Let's think about meal spacing here for a minute. If you sleep about eight hours each night (which I hope you do, and you'll see why in chapter 13), you have about sixteen hours each day to eat. When you skip or significantly delay breakfast, you cut into the number of hours available to distribute your meals. If you don't eat until noon, you're going to be hungry and cranky and make poor food choices. Waiting until you're ravenous to eat a meal is like waiting until you're drunk to drive. You'll make knuckleheaded decisions because your judgment is impaired. If you haven't consumed a majority of your food for the day before sitting down to dinner, fatness is soon to follow.

Still not sure eating breakfast is for you? Consider these facts:

- Breakfast helps us learn.[1] It's hard to memorize the essential amino acids when you don't have any of them floating around your bloodstream.
- Those who eat breakfast also make better food choices at lunch and dinner.[4, 9–11] Maybe it's because they have enough blood sugar to think with their brain instead of their gut.
- People who eat breakfast are more active.[9] I don't know about you, but I don't like to lift weights or do yoga when I feel like I'm about to pass out from hunger.

Planning for Success

Why is it that so many people wait for a grand finale dinner? My guess is lack of planning. If they prepared healthful, nutritious food in advance and had it available when they were hungry during the day, they'd probably eat more healthful foods and be leaner. But instead, they ignore hunger or try to satisfy it with nutritionally bankrupt convenience foods.

The bottom line? Plan ahead. And above all, don't skip breakfast. If you're too busy to eat a nutritious meal in the morning, you're too busy to be lean and healthy.

Chapter 2

Fat People Eat Haphazardly and Fast

Eat not ravenously, filling the mouth gulp after gulp without breathing space.

—Maimonides

As chapter 1 made abundantly evident, we know that fat people skip breakfast, and we have a sneaking suspicion that at 11:00 a.m. they don't recognize the error of their ways and adopt a regular eating schedule that stabilizes their blood sugar and keeps them energized for the rest of the day. It seems that big, infrequent meals are the norm for fat people. Heck, overweight people might even eat three or four huge meals at random times, and regardless of how often they eat, it's likely that they shovel their food down.

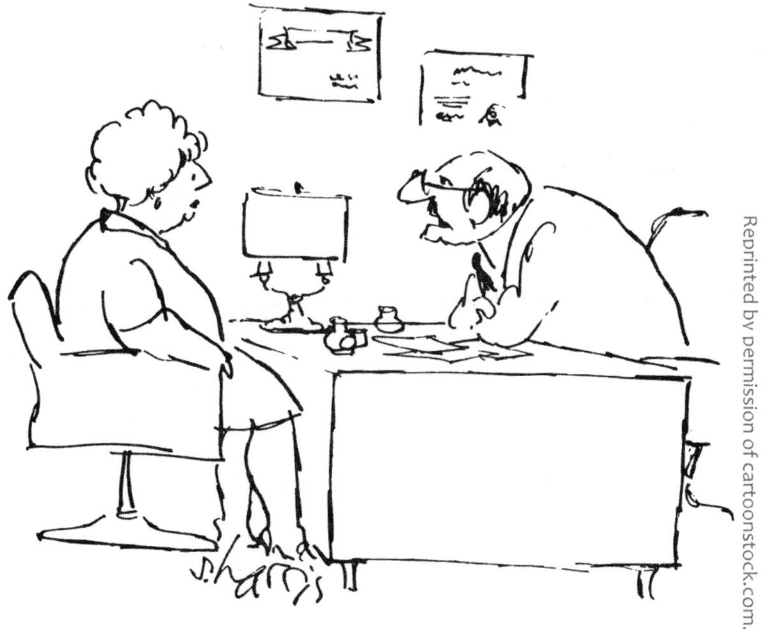

"It's partly glandular and partly 8,500 calories per day."

Sumo-Size Me

Here's the naked (and ugly) truth: random meals that are really big will make you not only fat, but also more likely to develop metabolic syndrome,[1] a condition that typically consists of high blood pressure, abdominal obesity, and high levels of cholesterol, triglycerides, and insulin and can lead to cardiovascular disease and diabetes.

If you aren't swayed by that harsh reality, or by my advice about haphazard meals, which is backed up by the opinions of countless experts, let's take a different approach. You're undoubtedly familiar with sumo wrestlers. Did you know that they typically aren't allowed to eat breakfast? In fact, they're instructed to eat huge, infrequent meals and drink a lot of calories (more on liquid calories in chapter 8). Why do they live this way? It isn't for a trim waistline and clean arteries; it's so they'll get fat—an advantage given that there aren't any weight divisions in sumo wrestling. To further maximize weight gain, they try to eat their biggest meal before going to sleep. Yet they're also more prone to diabetes, high blood pressure, and heart attacks and have a shorter life expectancy than the average Japanese man. So unless you're getting ready to enter the *dohyo* (ring) as a *rikishi* (wrestler), you might want to skip the sumo meal followed by a nap.

The advice to eat reasonably sized, frequent meals isn't exactly late-breaking news, and you may already have a good idea of some of the reasons to eat this way. Still, I'd like to highlight a few. For starters, when you eat regularly your body won't panic about when it's getting its next meal and drive you to eat to excess as an insurance policy. When you know you'll get your next meal in a few hours, it will be easier to forgo that extra sandwich.

A fundamental consideration is that the human body isn't built for huge feedings. We have a limited stomach capacity and a long gastrointestinal tract that digests food slowly, compared with animals that eat meat and gorge. Carnivorous animals have intestinal tracts that are three to six times their body length, while humans have intestinal tracts about twelve times our body length. The stomach capacity of humans is 21 to 27 percent of the total volume of our digestive tract, whereas for carnivorous animals it is 60 to 70 percent. It's no wonder that purely carnivorous animals can eat pounds and pounds of food in one sitting, taking in more than 25,000 calories solely from meat, or that lions can eat up to 25 percent of their body mass at one meal. After this meatfest, they won't eat again for a few days. But if we ate lion-style, we'd be forced to take lots of "food coma" naps. Plus, we'd be fat and miserable—not to mention that we'd rupture our stomachs.

Here's an idea: how about listening to the body's cues? Maybe you've heard the advice to eat when hungry and stop when no longer hungry. This may seem like an old-school approach in our world of twelve-hour workdays fueled by coffee, vending machine rations, and diet cola, but maybe it's time to get back to the basics. Lean people learn to listen to and heed physiological cues, including hunger—a vital biological signal that helps us seek our next feeding. And when they are no longer hungry, lean people stop eating. The best example of this is little kids who are still untainted by all of those media messages encouraging us to eat for the sake of eating or for some sort of life satisfaction. The appetite cues of little kids are pure. They want to eat when they're hungry, and they want to stop when they're satisfied.

You may have heard advice to eat five or six small meals a day. I'm not so sure that's a good idea. The data about this is mixed. Plenty of cultures stick to eating three times per day, and that seems works for most people. It also has the advantage of giving you fewer opportunities to think about food. The key here is to listen to your body. If eating three nutritious meals a day doesn't seem to satisfy you, try adding in some small, healthful snacks.

Why Speed Eating Isn't an Olympic Sport

I remember being at a concert and sitting next to a man who scarfed down a massive soft pretzel dipped in cheese sauce, a large slice of meat-laden pizza, and a jumbo cup of beer in less than six minutes. No matter what I thought of his food and beverage choices (gross), I was absolutely repulsed by how quickly he consumed them. It made me wonder: How often do fat people buy high-quality food, cook a healthful meal, and then set the table, turn off the TV, say a few words of thanks, and sit down to enjoy the meal with other people? My guess is not too often. Well, to be honest, it isn't a guess. I know it doesn't happen often because that's what fat clients tell me.

Fat and unhealthy people eat quickly.[2, 3] They have to because they're busy with other essential tasks, like watching reruns of *Celebrity Fit Club*, working long hours to pay off the flat-screen TV, and whining about not having time to go to the gym. Sorry, I know that sounds mean—but in my experience it's true.

Think about it: Would people be as fat if they actually thought about what they were eating and took the time to savor and enjoy their meals? People run into serious weight problems when they detach their experience of eating and simply shove food in their mouths while doing other things. I understand most people are stretched pretty thin these days, but recall the discussion in the introduction regarding what your schedule says about you. I challenge you to examine your life. If taking twenty minutes to eat a nutritious meal isn't near the top of your list, the rest of your life will suffer.

You may wonder if there's any science linking eating speed and fatness. There is. Let me introduce you to a hormone known by the glamorous name PYY(3-36), which travels from the gut to the brain to signal fullness.[4] It isn't exactly the Speedy Gonzales of hormones and tends to take at least twenty minutes to deliver its message. So a good way to control how much you eat is to slow down and take at least twenty minutes to eat your meal. This will allow a sense of satiety to kick in and let you know you're full.

A Timeless Solution

One of the most popular "new" behavioral approaches to weight control is eating mindfully. While mindfulness has its roots in ancient Buddhism, it isn't some arcane spiritual practice. Mindfulness simply means focusing on your present-moment experience. How cool is it that simply focusing on your meal instead of various distractions can help you get lean? Think about it: It's tough to focus on and enjoy a nice bowl of strawberries while watching reruns of *ER*. When you're eating, try to show respect for your food—and for your body—by focusing on eating. Maybe even take a minute to give thanks for the food.

When people eat while engaging in activities like watching TV, reading, working, using the Internet, or driving, food intake tends to go up, with body fat not far behind.[5–7] (In fact, it tends to end up very closely behind, if you know what I mean.) It probably doesn't come as a huge surprise that people seem to especially zone out and overeat while watching TV. In fact, one study showed that people who watched TV ate significantly more food than a similar group who listened to classical music.[8] What? You don't gorge on three huge bowls of mac and cheese while listening to Mozart? Weird. As for eating in the car, I think Victoria Moran put it best: "Eating in a car is like making love in a car: It is cramped, messy, and you're unlikely to respect yourself in the morning."[9]

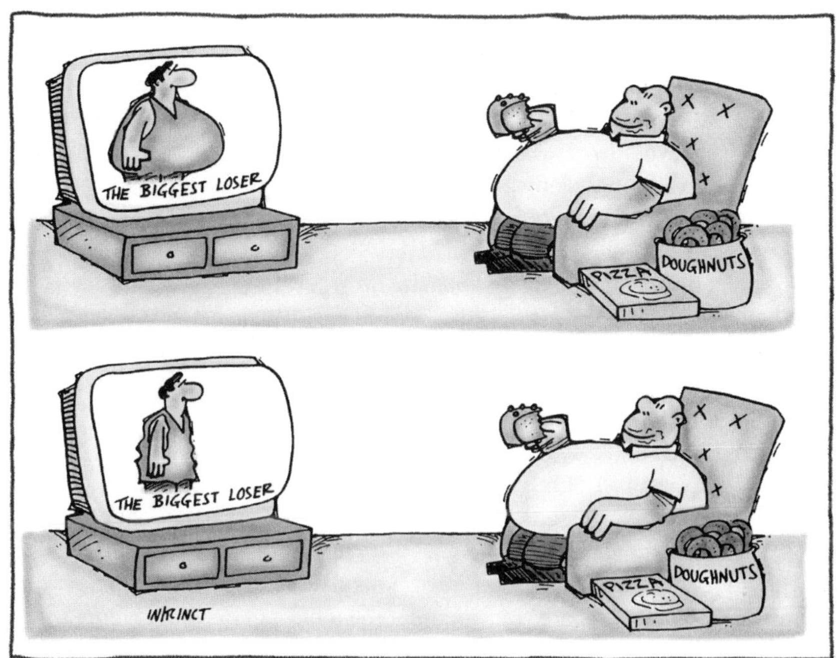

Thanks to John Ditchburn for this cartoon.

Eating mindfully is rapidly becoming a weight-loss cliché, but it holds merit. Simply put, it means actually being *present* for meals: smelling the food, feasting on it visually, appreciating its textures, savoring its flavors, chewing slowly, and generally enjoying it to the fullest. I think a lot of people tend to shovel down their food without noticing what they're doing, and then forget that they even ate. No wonder they think they're hungry again an hour or two later.

If you don't eat mindfully, you may take food for granted. As a result, it may be less satisfying and you'll find that you want to consume more. In addition, you may try to increase the level of stimulation you get from food. While eating can provide distraction and pleasure, these effects are only temporary. To keep these feelings going, you'll have to eat more, feeding a vicious cycle.

I can already hear you whining: "But Ryan, eating is so *boring*. I want to watch TV while I eat." Isn't this just one of countless desires that crop up each day? Maybe you want to show up late for work, tell off your boss, or just skip work altogether. Maybe you don't want to pay your bills this month or yield the right-of-way. Heck, maybe you want to bear false witness, steal, and commit adultery. We all have less-than-noble impulses. And if everyone acted on these desires, the world would be in complete anarchy.

There are good reasons for having rules, including those you set up for yourself. Think of it as sort of like becoming your own parent. Hopefully your parents gave you some basic rules for healthful living. Assuming that you aren't still living in your folks' basement and toeing their line, you need to take responsibility for establishing your own rules. Here are some of the rules I set for myself that I recommend to all of my clients. While they may seem restrictive, with time you'll realize how much more you're enjoying your meals—not to mention good health, and life in general:

- Don't eat while reading or watching TV.
- Don't eat while driving.
- Sit down at a table to eat.
- Don't eat dessert before dinner.
- Eat your vegetables.
- Go outside and play with friends.
- Don't stay up all night.
- If you want to buy something, you'd better have enough money in your piggy bank to pay for it.

To sum things up, here's my recommendation for the ultimate way to approach mealtime: Prepare your food, set the table, put on your favorite music or sit across from someone whose company you enjoy, give thanks for the food, then savor the meal and eat at a leisurely pace. Give it a try. It's a very pleasurable strategy for getting lean.

Chapter 3
Fat People Count Calories

Avoiding adequate calories actually promotes eating disturbances and weight gain. . . . Quality calories are good for you. When you eat enough, they keep you from craving, and bingeing on, lousy food.

—Jean Antonello, RN, BSN

I'm always amazed to discover that people are still counting calories. In my view, this approach is primarily effective for developing stress, anxiety, and a preoccupation with food. Focusing on consuming only a certain number of calories creates an experience of restriction and limitation. If this is you, once you hit X number of calories for the day you'll think you must stop eating. It doesn't matter whether you're hungry, jet-lagged, sick, or training for the national shuffleboard championships.

Many people believe that they're 100 percent in control when they count calories, but I think they're fooling themselves. It's hard to outsmart a biological system honed by eons of evolution, in which the brain regulates food intake and energy balance based on information from neural connections, hormone receptors, and sensory data about nutrient availability at the cellular level—messages that are based on energy depletion, time of day, physical activity level, developmental stage, stressors, food supply, and a number of other factors.[1]

In my experience, the most assiduous calorie counters tend to be overweight and unhealthy and have a miserable relationship with food. (Well, to be honest, some of them are malnourished and underweight.) Even though I'm a nutritionist, these folks typically have more knowledge about the number of calories in specific foods than I do. Yet they keep overeating.

In contrast, the healthiest and leanest people I've known don't count calories. They simply have calorie awareness. They know that chicken fried steak, chili cheese fries, and lemon meringue pie are calorie-dense. They also know that veggies, fruits, whole grains, and legumes are less calorie-dense, while also providing a host of nutrients, including plenty of fiber (which helps you feel more full and keeps you feeling satisfied for a longer time). More importantly, fit people focus on quality of food rather than quantity and listen to their fullness cues.

Keeping Your Eye on the Doughnut

I find that when people focus excessively on calories, they often lose sight of the importance of eating enough health-promoting food. Here's a glimpse at how this might play out:

Me: "How is your nutrition going?"

Client: "Well, I didn't exceed my calorie quota yesterday!"

Me: "Okay, so what did you actually eat?"

Client: "A double-bacon cheeseburger and a chocolate malt."

Me: "Congratulations on your poor nutrition. I'll put your sticker in the mail."

This focus on calories, often leads to a fixation on calorie-dense but nutritionally void foods: the burgers, bacon, cheese, cookies, and doughnuts that fat people don't want to give up. It's no wonder they can't stay lean. When I focus on ice cream, I end up spending a lot of time thinking about ice cream—and then getting a craving for it. Fit people take a different tack: they focus on the nutritious foods they plan to eat.

Maybe fat people are approaching calorie counting like money management. After all, if you want to be financially fit and save money for the future, you need to create a detailed budget and account for where all of your money goes. Hmm, but last I checked the average American household carried about $8,000 in credit card debt and about 43 percent of families spend more money than they earn each year.[2]

So Americans tend to suck at money management, and I have to tell you: the body is a lot more complicated than your checkbook—as are calories. The calorie is actually a fairly abstract concept, and all calories aren't equal.

A Calorie Is Just a Calorie—or Is It?

I can hear you now: "Hold on a minute! Did you just say that all calories aren't equal?" Don't break into a cold sweat or go fainting on me. Take a deep breath, and when you've calmed down a bit, let me explain.

Are you ready to hear the news that the diet and packaged-food industries absolutely don't want you to know? Processing and refining foods tends to make their calories more available, whereas the body has to work harder to extract the calories locked into fiber-rich whole foods.[3] If you're an old-school dieter, you may already be at least a little familiar with this. Maybe you've looked at celery as an excellent snack because you heard you burn more calories chewing celery than the celery itself contains. Folks, you'd have to approach chewing as an Olympic sport for this to be true. However, because the body expends calories at all phases of the digestive process, celery actually does contain so-called negative calories. Simply put, it takes more calories to digest celery than you actually obtain from the celery. Do I recommend an all-celery diet? Of course not.

Still, this celery example does a good job of illustrating the fact that the digestive process has an impact on how many net calories you obtain from various foods. For similar reasons, the net amount of calories available from fiber-rich whole grains is less than the amount available from the same grains once they're processed and the bran has been removed.

Another factor that often has an even larger effect on available calories is cooking. Heat changes the structure of starches and proteins, making it easier for digestive enzymes to access them and break them down into smaller components that are more readily absorbed by the body.[3]

There are a couple of take-away messages here. The first is that, as usual, Mother Nature knows best. Eating the foods she provides, in their natural forms, can go a long way toward keeping you lean and healthy. I'm not saying you have to eat an entirely raw, whole-food diet. But the more you incorporate these kinds of foods into your diet, the better.

The second take-away message is to be skeptical of calorie counts on food labels. Realize that your body is probably going to reap every last calorie from a conventional sugary breakfast cereal (and put it right on your hips), as opposed to a minimally sweetened granola. So which is it going to be?

Why Do We Believe What We Believe?

I often wonder why we believe what we believe, especially after I see something like an ad claiming that breakfast sausage will help improve my energy levels all day. What!?

In interactions with clients (and anyone, really), I find that people have some deep-rooted beliefs regarding what they eat and how they exercise. And I'm always curious about why people believe what they believe. Did they read it in a magazine? Did they learn it from their parents? Did they see it on a TV commercial? Did they research it for a thesis project? Did they use outcome-based decision making and find out if it worked for their lifestyle? Did they read it on a fortune cookie label? And do any of these methods really hold more weight than others?

Shifting Focus

If you're legitimately hungry and you've already met your calorie quota for the day, should you really stop eating? You may find it hard to believe, but my recommendation is that you go ahead and eat more. Your body apparently needs more nutrition. The catch here is that you need to eat real food, and you need to stop short of feeling stuffed. If a bowl of squash and pinto beans doesn't sound good but a cookie does, then it probably isn't true hunger; it's just a craving.

We don't tend to frequently eat healthful whole foods to excess. Have you ever just kept eating and eating from a pot of plain quinoa or chickpeas? What about licking your fingers after eating a boiled yam while hovered over the sink? Have you ever stuffed handfuls of kale in your mouth while standing in front of an open fridge? I didn't think so. The take-home message? Instead of fixating on numbers, focus on eating unprocessed, whole foods. This will regulate your appetite and break fat-promoting feast-and-famine cycles.

Chapter 4
Fat People Go on Diets

The road to hell is paved with good intentions.

—Proverb

If I asked you what the best weight-loss strategy is, would you say dieting, or perhaps cutting out certain foods? If so, I have bad news for you: following a restricted diet may give you a sense of control or effectiveness, but it doesn't seem to lead to long-term leanness. In fact, it tends to backfire and cause overeating. There are a few key reasons for this: physiological realities, psychological cravings, and disappointment when results aren't immediate. Let's examine the last one first.

Seeking Immediate Gratification

One day on my way home from the gym, I noticed two scratch cards (already scratched) and a nickel lying on the sidewalk. My investigative skills helped me piece together the sequence of events: Someone bought the scratch cards, pulled out a nickel, scratched the cards, didn't win, got pissed, and threw everything on the sidewalk. Isn't that the American way? Someone hopes to score the $50,000 jackpot and doesn't think twice about wasting $2.05 in the process ($2 for the cards and a nickel to scratch them).

This is the mind-set at work when people start a new diet and then give up when they don't get results in two weeks. Here's an idea: how about cultivating a lifelong practice of eating nutritious foods and exercising a few times each week? While fat people keep starting new diets and then giving up on them, fit people achieve long-term success by plugging away at reasonable, effective behaviors.

Folks, I hate to be the bearer of bad news, but you won't get a tight waistline after a day or a week of eating healthfully. Depending on where you're starting from, it may take months. In the meanwhile, you have to trust your approach and keep the long-term outcome in mind.

That probably sounds reasonable enough, at least in theory. Yet we live in a world where people with all the money, resources, trainers, chefs, and incentive to get lean and stay lean can't do it, including celebrities, public figures, and even the people on weight-loss reality shows (okay, maybe that last one isn't such a surprise).

Of course, the pull of immediate gratification plays into the fatness equation in other ways too. Here's a test: After a long day of work—maybe one where you skipped lunch—walk by a bakery and take a good, long whiff. Then go home and read this book. I'm guessing that the lure of freshly baked treats exerted a stronger pull. The hardest part of living a fit lifestyle may well be resisting the desire for immediate gratification.

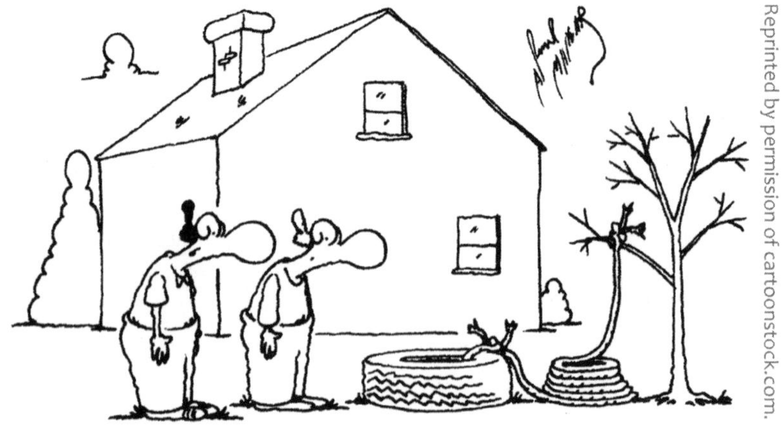

"My parents are trying to wean me off instant gratification."

Cultivating a Negative Energy Balance

Many people say they want to look like bodybuilders. And if you're serious about getting ready for the state championships, a rigid meal plan will be your best friend (at least in the short term). But bear in mind that I used to be a competitive bodybuilder and trust me when I tell you that bodybuilders don't look as ripped in day-to-day life as they do in pictures. They only look totally picture-worthy for about twelve hours. Care to hazard a guess as to what most bodybuilders look forward to doing the minute their photos have been taken? Eating something not on the meal plan.

A planned reduction of food intake *can* lead to weight loss and a buff body. But it does so by creating a negative energy balance—and that doesn't happen in isolation. Your body doesn't just burn fat; it also experiences hunger, moodiness, altered sleep patterns, and more. And here's the kicker: When control of eating shifts from physiological (governed by the energy needs of our cells) to cognitive (governed by strong intellectual urges), any sort of agitation (stress, family concerns, overwork, deviation from your daily routine, and so forth) can lead to out-of-control eating. This cycle can get ugly—fast. Which leads me to my next point: psychological craving.

Ensuring Maximum Cravings

Here's a meal plan I'd like you to consider. Check it out and see how it strikes you:

Breakfast: 4 scrambled egg whites and oatmeal made from ½ cup oats.

Lunch: 5 ounces of broiled skinless chicken with ½ cup steamed broccoli.

Snack: 1 piece of fruit and 10 walnuts.

Dinner: A large green salad with ½ cup pinto beans and 2 tablespoons hempseeds.

On the surface, this might look like the recipe for an effective weight-loss program. It even has the advantage of focusing primarily on nutrient-dense and mostly whole foods. So what's the problem? If you try to eat this way day in, day out, it might make you fat. Sure, it looks great when plugged into a spreadsheet, but that doesn't translate into working well for the body—much less the mind. Folks, I hate to break it to you, but here's how a repetitious, restricted diet actually plays out for most people:

Breakfast: 4 scrambled egg whites and oatmeal made from ½ cup oats.

Breakfast B: If your breakfast leaves you feeling restricted and deprived, your body, your brain, or both will retaliate. Next thing you know, you're stopping at a bakery for a triple mocha and a muffin. No, wait! Make that two muffins.

Lunch: 5 ounces of broiled skinless chicken with ½ cup steamed broccoli, ½ cup barbecue sauce or salsa, a dollop of fat-free sour cream, a liberal dousing of low-fat fake butter spray, and a jumbo diet soda, because, gosh, those are all "free" foods, right?

Snack: 1 piece of fruit and 10 walnuts.

Snack B: Your snack wasn't very satisfying because you didn't eat what you wanted. Plus, work is kind of slow and you're bored. Before you realize it, you've cleared out the candy dish at the receptionist's desk, and that granola bar from the vending machine is starting to sound pretty tasty.

Dinner: A large green salad with ½ cup pinto beans and 2 tablespoons hempseeds.

Late-night food fest: Not only was your dinner boring, everything on TV is dull—except the advertisements for food. It's late, you're tired, and your guard is down. You figure that you already blew it today, so you might as well cave in, get the cravings out of your system, and start your diet again tomorrow. Besides, you've only got "health-promoting" snack food on hand, so it's not so bad. Next stop: the pantry for three handfuls of "lean" jerky nuggets, a bowl of "all natural" trail mix, a slice of bread with butter, and, oh sure, why not, some reduced-fat potato chips. Still, you crave a little something sweet, and surely eating a few spoonfuls of "lite" ice cream in front of the freezer doesn't count—especially if you're the only one who knows that you managed to cram half a pint into those spoonfuls.

Curses, Foiled Again!

Many clients tell me their biggest barrier is a flawed meal plan—a diet that just doesn't seem to deliver what it promises. Guess again. The problem is all of the extra foods they conveniently overlook: cheesy puffs eaten while hovering over the sink, the remnants of other family members' dinners, the slice (or two, or three) of brownie "just to even up the edges." Meanwhile, these folks are blaming that darned meal plan: it must be those walnuts—or maybe that piece of fruit.

Once people give in to the desire to eat without restrictions, they either feel guilty or gain weight—or both. So they end up wanting to restrict their eating even further, which only increases the chances of more binge eating. Plus, binge eating often leads to higher levels of dopamine, which is tied in with the brain's reward system. Not surprisingly, we tend to repeat behaviors associated with rewards. If you stay on this roller coaster for too long, it will destroy your relationship with eating.

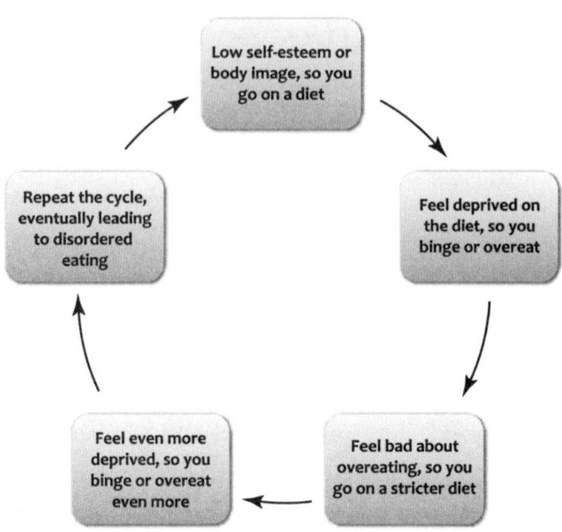

Still not convinced that strict diets may actually predict fatness? Then just consider the hard, cold facts:

- One study found that dietary restraint and radical weight control behaviors can predict the onset of obesity in adolescent girls.[1]
- Another study showed that higher levels of dietary restraint, obsessions about weight, and body dissatisfaction were accompanied by greater weight gain in girls as young as five to nine years old.[2]
- Other studies indicate that children and adolescents who diet are at increased risk of being overweight later.[3,4]

Obeying One Rule of a Fat Stomach

The hazards of restrictive diets even apply to following well-intentioned nutritional advice for eating well. Sound counterintuitive? Let me explain.

Let's say you read on a website that you should eat carbs only after exercising. The science behind this recommendation seems sound, so you decide to make this one of your dietary rules. But rules are, by definition, inflexible, and that's where the problem arises. Now imagine this scenario: It's dinnertime on a typical weeknight and you exercised during your lunch hour—or, time to fess up, maybe you didn't exercise at all that day. Either way, your rule says you can't have any carbs with your evening meal, even though you really want some rice. You suck it up, tell yourself no, and decide to have steamed veggies and grilled tempeh.

You feel virtuous and everything seems fine and dandy . . . until the end of the meal, when you still feel hungry. You feel short-changed because you didn't get that rice. So you decide to have an after-dinner snack. Once again you rule out carb-dense foods and opt for nuts and berries. A cup of almonds and a pint of berries later you feel good about yourself for staying compliant, but you're still thinking about that rice. Fast-forward to two weeks later: you're probably feeling frustrated that you still aren't seeing any changes in body composition.

Now let's look at an alternative: What if you originally had a side of brown rice with your veggies and tempeh that night for dinner? Whole-grain rice has plenty of fiber, which would have helped you feel full, and it also contains good amounts of minerals and B vitamins, and even some protein. If you'd eaten the rice, maybe you would have actually felt content and satisfied with the meal. Instead, you felt deprived and ended up eating a massive amount of almonds and berries. While this is a very nutritious combination, it adds up to a lot of fat, sugars, and, yes, even calories. While I'm not a fan of counting calories, I'm not naive, and neither are you. The energy you consume is either used by the body or stored for a later time (translation: becomes body fat).

This is just one among endless possible rules for healthful eating. Maybe you think you shouldn't eat bananas; maybe you think a small cup of yogurt is a sufficient breakfast; maybe you think fat-free foods are the answer. It's truth time. Is the way you've been approaching nutrition rules working for you? I honestly believe that the best strategy for achieving your health and body composition goals isn't going to be any single rule or new diet fad. The answer is to find a food strategy that you can stick with, one that helps you satisfy your body's hunger and manage your psychological cravings.

Dieting Do's and Don'ts: Just Don't Do It

It may be hard to let go of the idea that dieting is the answer, especially with the constant harping on that theme in books and magazines. One of the best things I ever did for my health was *decrease* the time I spent reading fitness magazines. After years of reading them, I started feeling overwhelmed and frustrated. There was too much conflicting advice and too many magic diet plans. The Internet is even worse. (And, please, don't tell me you've never been tempted to believe that one weird, old, or simple trick could give you a flat belly.)

Talk about information overload! My recommendation? Stick with straightforward information and don't confuse yourself with fads and hype.

Let's revisit the analogy of money management. Many people feel like their money woes would be alleviated if they would just set up the right budget. Yet nearly half of American families spend more than they earn each year, and the average household carries major debt. People typically follow strict line-item budgets about as well as they follow rigid, repetitive meal plans.

What's the secret of the financially fit? Well, one thing they *don't* do is create unrealistic budgets and then retaliate with overspending. Right now, take a minute to realistically assess how you've responded to rigid meal plans in the past. Have they worked for you? If not, consider the following alternatives.

- **Set reasonable limits on eating.** If you have kids, think about how you try to guide them in regard to eating. You don't put them on a strict diet or rigid meal plan (at least I hope you don't). But you also probably don't let them have dessert every night or stand in front of the refrigerator drinking a quart of chocolate milk.
- **Avoid both restrictions and cheating.** Eat healthful foods that you enjoy, and eat them in reasonable amounts. Take some time to listen to the feedback your body is providing. If you feel a bit bloated, you probably ate too much. If you feel deprived, you may be avoiding too many foods that you like. If you're obsessed with your next meal, you probably aren't eating enough nutritious food.
- **Eat a reasonable amount of quality food each day, forever.** Rather than being attached to the idea that diets, rules, and meal plans are the best way to control weight, try to develop a healthy relationship with food and your body. Make reasonable, rational choices every day. Purposefully choose foods that nourish and sustain you, savor them as you consume them, and toss the restrictive diet plans in the trash, along with the low-fat fake butter spray. If you do this, you'll have the body you were meant to.

Chapter 5
Fat People Eat Processed Foods

Clearly, some time ago makers and consumers of American junk food passed jointly through some kind of sensibility barrier in the endless quest for new taste sensations. Now they are a little like those desperate junkies who have tried every known drug and are finally reduced to mainlining toilet bowl cleanser in an effort to get still higher.

—Bill Bryson

Pop quiz: What's the best appetite suppressant?

The answer? Food. But before you rush out the door to the local fast-food drive-through, please read on. I'm talking about *real* food. And maybe even more importantly, I'm talking about real appetite. Fake, processed foods won't keep you feeling satisfied for very long after you've eaten them.

So many overweight people complain about having a ravenous appetite. I'm not surprised after I look at what they eat:

- Sugary cereal with skim milk for breakfast
- A granola bar or crackers with nonfat fruit-flavored yogurt for a mid-morning snack
- A sandwich on "wheat" bread with low-fat cheese and deli meat (read: animal flesh pumped full of carcinogenic preservatives) for lunch
- A microwave "diet meal" for dinner

If any of those sound like the next meal you intend to eat, you might be better off passing, no matter how ravenous you are. Here's hoping the nutrition fairy grants you some good sense by the time the next meal rolls around. What's the common theme? Processed and pathetic. There's no real food being consumed. I'd be hungry after eating this way too.

If I read the ingredient list on a food product and it sounds like a chemistry experiment, I know it isn't a real food, and I'm definitely not going to eat it. I encourage you not to eat it either, at least not on a regular basis. Instead, opt for real food: vegetables, fruits, beans and other legumes, nuts and seeds, and whole grains. While I don't eat meat, eggs, or dairy products, I do recognize that for some people these can be "real" foods too—but not if they come from animals raised on factory farms or in feedlots. And, of course, no animal products are necessary to sustain health (and most animal-based foods tend to do just the opposite, regardless of how the animals are raised).

The sad fact is, most of what passes for food these days is anything but. Real food makes up less than 1 percent of the forty-five thousand items at the typical supermarket.[1] Because real food typically doesn't make companies loads of profit, it isn't usually advertised on TV (which is where most people seem to get their menu ideas). That's a shame, because real food has a lot going for it. If you haven't tried any lately, give it a whirl. You just might find that it tastes good, and that you don't feel compelled to keep eating it until you're overstuffed. Better yet, you're likely to find that it makes you lean, healthy, and happy. And perhaps best of all, it's more sustainable for the planet.

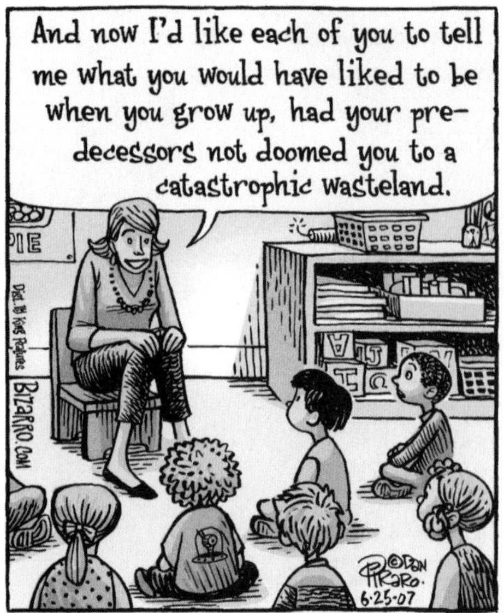

And now I'd like each of you to tell me what you would have liked to be when you grow up, had your predecessors not doomed you to a catastrophic wasteland.
PIE
BIZARRO.COM
©DON PIRARO. 6-25-07
Bizarro, reprinted by permission of Dan Piraro.

The Devil Isn't in the Details

Are you sitting down? I'm about to drop a bombshell: It doesn't matter if you follow a more meat-oriented paleo diet, stick strictly to plant-based foods, or are a flexitarian, sometimes eating meat and sometimes going veggie. If you're healthy, fit, and lean—and have been for a while—I bet you eat much like I do.

People who adhere to or advocate various diets tend to claim that their diet is *drastically* different and *drastically* better than others. I think they're ignoring the big picture: a variety of diets can be health promoting, and all of them have more similarities than differences. If you set out a day's worth of food for any healthy, fit person, the graphic on the following page shows what you probably would see.

Typically, the differences between various healthful diets is minimal and occurs mainly in that 15 percent or so of food in the category that consists of legumes, meat, fish, eggs, or dairy products. Other than that, people with healthful eating habits consume essentially the same foods.

So where do people go wrong? How is a fat or unfit person's diet different? It comes down to the proportion of what I call "degenerate foods": processed grains, meat, and soy products; refined sweeteners; artificial ingredients; and so forth. Here's what it looks like:

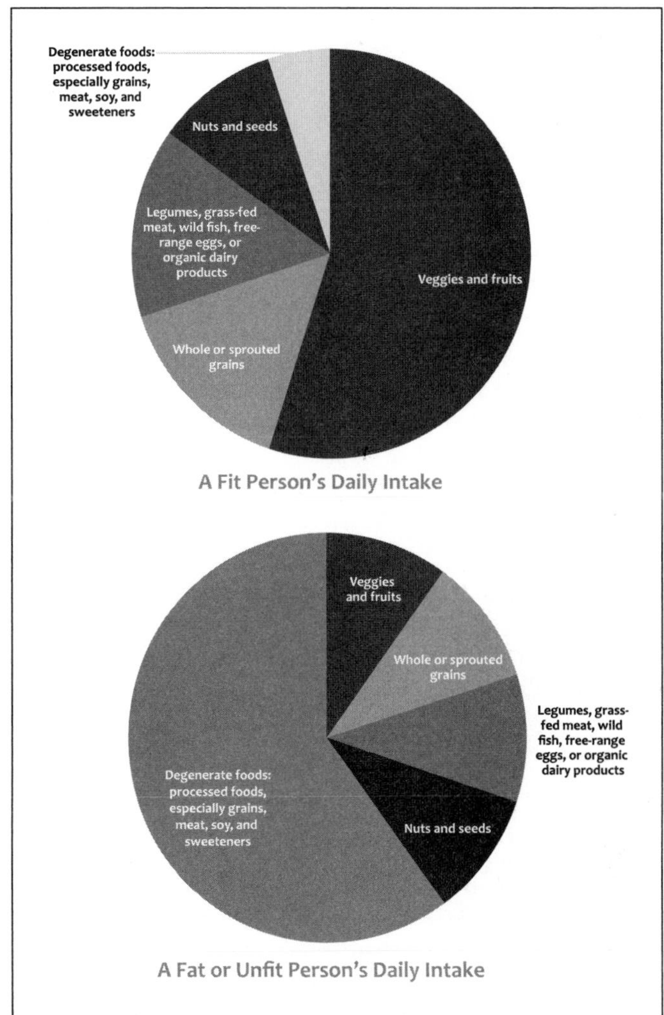

The Devil *Is* in Refined Grains

Whole grains are currently getting a lot of good press for their health benefits—accompanied by the inevitable barrage of marketing that occurs whenever the next healthy food fad comes along. (Not that I'm saying whole grains are a fad; in fact, learning how to cultivate grains was a key factor in the rise of various ancient civilizations.) While many people at least claim to be interested in eating more whole grains, there's a lot of confusion regarding exactly what qualifies as a whole grain, and that can get in the way of good intentions. Given that sugary cereals with marshmallows tout their whole-grain goodness these days, this confusion is understandable.

It's time for a vocabulary lesson. "Deceptive," "mysterious," "misleading," and "illusory"—these four words don't just describe your ex; they also describe many of the claims you'll find on food packaging. I often wonder if reading the front of a box of cereal—or most any other type of packaged food—provides any helpful information at all. When I read the more outrageous claims, I'm baffled. I'd like to think most people know that good nutrition doesn't start with sandwich cookies and cheese-flavored crackers. But apparently many people buy these claims. So in case you had any doubt, let me clear something up: 100-calorie packs aren't a real solution to the problems with most people's diets. There's just no comparing the grains or nutrients in those 100-calorie packs to a serving of home-cooked quinoa.

Food manufacturers generally want consumers to think health and weight management come down to controlling portion sizes and being more physically active. That way they can continue to sell lots of crappy food. They don't want you to think about the merits of particular foods. After all, if people actually ate foods that contributed to health and weight management, the term "sandwich cookie" wouldn't be part of our vocabulary.

There are several reasons why you don't generally see vegetables, fruits, legumes, whole grains, nuts, and seeds offered in packaging with lots of splashy claims about their health benefits. Any guess as to the biggest reason? It's because there typically isn't a lot of money to be made by selling these humble but highly nutritious foods.

To trademark and patent their products and thus reap higher profits, manufacturers create strange new foodstuffs that should more accurately be considered nonfoods. While quite a few convenience foods are grain based, those poor grains are tortured all along the way, being ground up, denatured, and mixed with processed fats, sweeteners, and artificial ingredients before finally being extruded and fried into submission. Unfortunately, this processing leaves the "food" nutritionally bankrupt. Still, these products have a draw, and when that's combined with dubious health claims emblazoned on the packaging, many people (fat people) find themselves reaching for processed foods, including those infernal 100-calorie packs. I might as well go ahead and get on my soapbox, since I obviously have a beef with 100-calorie packs. Sure, they might seem like a moderate choice, but that's mainly because manufacturers slap their own health logos on the packaging so consumers are duped into thinking a nutritious food lurks inside. But not only do these portioned packs contain all of the evils of processed former foods, they also feed into an entire culture of fatness, wherein the mountains of discarded packaging from these products of convenience bloat our landfills. Not good.

Gosh, I really meant to get down off my soapbox, but as long as I'm up here . . . *Processed foods make me crazy!* Hmm, or maybe it's human gullibility that makes me crazy. Here's the situation: I was listening to the radio and an ad came on with testimonials from parents praising an amazing new time-saving snack. The wonder food being proffered? Frozen peanut butter and jelly pocket sandwiches, which save precious seconds of sandwich-making time. Seriously? If people can't buy a loaf of bread and jars of peanut butter and jelly to construct one of the most basic sandwich combinations in human history for their kids, they need to reevaluate their priorities. When I hear this kind of stuff, I'm surprised that Americans aren't fatter and more diseased than they already are.

Keepin' It Real

Let's continue with our vocabulary lesson. Strictly speaking, "whole grain" simply means that nothing has been stripped from the grain. Whole-grain products contain the bran, germ, and endosperm of the grain. "Refined," on the other hand, means components of the grain have been removed. White flour is the classic example of a refined grain product. Both the bran and the germ have been removed, and with them 80 percent of the fiber and 30 percent of the protein. But here's an interesting point: seemingly healthful products like oat bran, wheat bran, and wheat germ can also be considered to be refined, as they are just single components of the entire grain and therefore don't offer the full nutritional benefits of whole grains.

I think it's also important to include the word "processed" in this vocabulary lesson. As evil as it sounds, it does include simply grinding whole grains into flour. However, in my view, the only form of grain that truly qualifies as a whole grain is, in fact, whole: brown rice, oat and barley groats, wheat berries, and whole amaranth, millet, quinoa, and so on. Don't get me wrong; Whole-grain breads, crackers, pasta, and other foods made with whole-grain flour are a much better choice than their counterparts made with refined flour. However, they still aren't optimal. That said, I understand that most folks will want to eat foods like bread, crackers, and pasta in some form or another. When you do so, try to opt for products made with sprouted whole grains. While these processed foods still are not ideal, sprouting greatly boosts the nutrients in the grains, so these products are nutritionally superior to similar ones made with unsprouted whole grains.

Looking for Whole Grains in All the Wrong Places

Many people want to believe they can incorporate sufficient quantities of whole grains into their diet without hitting up the oats, quinoa, millet, or sprouted-grain breads. A classic place to pursue this pipe dream is in the supermarket bread aisle. Perhaps you feel virtuous about purchasing breads "made with whole grains." Unfortunately, the whole-grain content of these breads is typically 30 percent or less. (Still, if the choice is that or white bread, they are a very minor improvement.) Even worse, most products labeled "multigrain," "seven-grain," or "wheat" are actually worthless in terms of whole-grain content.

And if you're hoping to meet your whole-grain quota by eating out, think again. On average, 1,000 calories of restaurant food provides less than 0.4 ounce of whole grains,[2] whereas the recommended intake is more in the range of 3.5 ounces. Time for a reality check: You'd have to eat about 10,000 calories of restaurant food to meet your whole-grain goal for the day.

A true whole-grain food should list one of the following as its first ingredient:

- amaranth
- barley
- brown rice
- bulgur
- corn
- Kamut
- millet
- oats
- quinoa
- whole rye
- whole wheat
- wild rice

It doesn't take that much effort to include two to three servings of whole grains in your diet each day. For example, you could have oatmeal for breakfast, a sandwich on sprouted-grain bread at lunch, and a side of quinoa or brown rice with dinner to meet your quota.

The Wonderful World of Fiber

Brace yourself for some bad news: On average, Americans consume only about 15 grams of fiber daily.[3] Folks, I eat that much before 8:00 a.m. Ideally you should be consuming well over twice that amount daily, and eating more unprocessed food is one excellent way to achieve this.

What makes fiber so beneficial? More bad news: We're going to have to talk about bowel movements, even though this isn't a popular topic. Fiber helps add bulk to the stool and makes it easier for digested food to travel through your gut. Lack of fiber, on the other hand, is a recipe for fatness, not to mention chronic constipation and bowel-related illnesses, including diverticulosis and cancer.[3,4] The good news? If you build your diet around whole, natural foods—fruits, legumes, nuts, seeds, vegetables, and whole grains—you definitely won't need to tally up your fiber intake on an abacus. You'll be getting enough. As one major study of nearly twenty-one thousand people put it, "Being vegetarian and especially vegan is strongly associated with a higher frequency of bowel movements."[5] Don't you just love science?

But as mentioned, the United States is a nation of fiber degenerates. That probably explains why powdered fiber supplements seem to get as much attention as the NFL playoffs. Many people have become reliant upon these fiber supplements to achieve their "daily constitutional."

I thought powdered fiber supplements were bad enough. Then one day I discovered a sample of an artificial sweetener with added fiber in my mailbox. No freakin' way! Are we seriously at a point where people have been convinced that this is a good way to add fiber to their diets? Newsflash: There is an amazing variety of colorful natural foods that happen to have a sweet flavor *and* be packed with fiber. They are known as fruits. Ta-da! I suggest that you invest in an orange—unless you're in the market for a synthetic sweetener that creates disordered eating habits, promotes overconsumption of other foods, and potentially leads to cancer and neurological disorders.[6–9]

1.6 Ounces of Prevention Is Worth . . .

Let's look at how easy it is to get enough fiber. Here's a sample day of eating, excluding dinner:

Food	Fiber (grams)
Breakfast shake (made with frozen fruit, kale, almond milk, hempseed protein, flaxseeds, cacao nibs, and a bit of supplemental greens powder)	12
Cooked quinoa	5
Carrots, sugar snap peas, and hummus	5
Sprouted-grain bread and nut butter	8
Green salad with black beans	12
Apple	4
Total	46

That's 46 grams, or 1.6 ounces, all before dinner!

Since we're on the topic of fiber and bowel movements, I need to briefly mention water. Staying well hydrated is good for you in so many ways, including facilitating regular bowel movements. Beware of eating too much fiber and not drinking enough water. Okay, thanks for sticking with me through this discussion of bowel issues. I know it may seem unsavory, but you'll thank me in fifteen years when your doctor doesn't leave you a voice mail regarding severe diverticulitis.

But hey, let's end this discussion on a more upbeat note. While I hope you care more about your health than a number on a scale, this is a book about weight loss. And guess what? Eating more fiber means eating more bulk, and eating more bulk means a fuller, happier stomach—with fewer calories. If you want to feel more full and satisfied and keep feeling that way longer, eating more fiber-rich foods is the way to go.

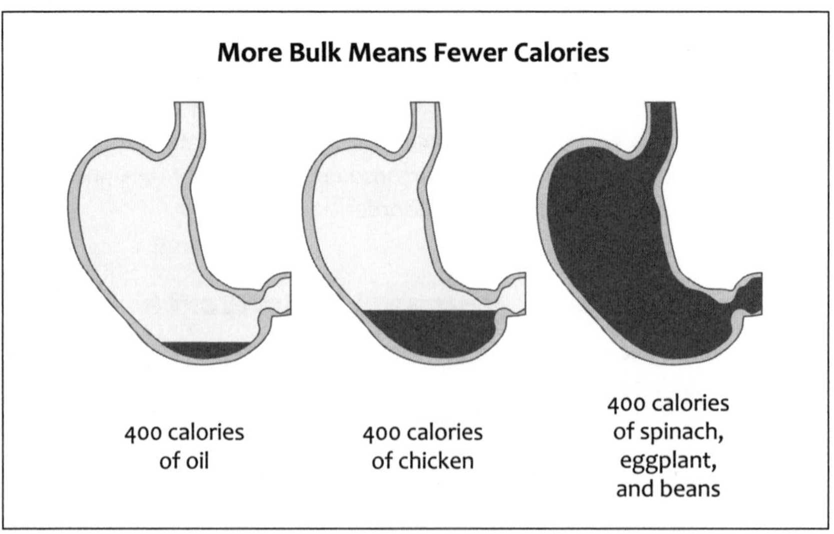

Reprinted from *Eat to Live* by permission of Joel Fuhrman, MD (drfuhrman.com).

Tasty versus Too Tasty

I like food that's tasty. I don't like food that's *too tasty*. When I think of food that's too tasty, I think of processed food and refined grains, and as you'll recall from my time up on the soapbox, those kinds of foods make me loco!

Back in my early high school years, I used to eat fast food all the time. That stuff was so tasty that I didn't want to stop eating it. Even when I physically felt full, for some reason I wanted to keep eating. I'm guessing that you've experienced this too. Here are some examples, based on my experience.

Tasty: raw, unsalted nut butter. (It's simple, satisfying, and tasty.)
Too tasty: salted nut butter with sugar added. (That's way too much stimulation for my taste buds.)

Tasty: brown rice and veggie stir-fry made at home. (After one plate, I'm set.)
Too tasty: rice and veggie stir-fry from the local Chinese take-out. (After one plate, I'm ready for five more. Let's hear it for poor-quality oil and MSG!)

Tasty: raw, unsalted nuts or seeds. (A few handfuls and I'm content.)
Too tasty: roasted, salted, and sweetened or flavored nuts. (Better get the wholesale-size container so I have enough to last me for a few days.)

Tasty: a baked potato or sweet potato. (It's tasty and satisfying.)
Too tasty: french fries and potato chips. (After eating just a few, I don't want any more. . . . Wait a minute—yeah, I do.)

Tasty: sprouted-grain bread. (A slice of this stuff with hummus or nut butter and I'm good to go.)
Too tasty: white flour breads. (So light! So fluffy! I think I'll have three or four more pieces!)

Tasty: fruit. (If I eat two pieces of whole fruit, I'm sated.)
Too tasty: dried fruit (Gosh, that was a five-pound bag?)

Tasty: buckwheat, oatmeal, polenta, quinoa, wild rice, or almost any cooked whole grain. (After one bowl, I'm not looking for more.)
Too tasty: standard cold breakfast cereals with added sugars and chemistry-experiment ingredients. (In junior high I spent way too many days with "sugar bloat" after eating endless bowls of the stuff.)

Tasty: homemade raw cookies with dates, walnuts, and coconut. (I feel satisfied after just one or two.)
Too tasty: cookies made with white flour, margarine or oil, and refined sweeteners. (The combination of oil, flour, and sweetener makes for taste overload and addictive eating.)

Tasty: cooked whole beans. (One of nature's perfect foods, beans are supremely satisfying.)
Too tasty: refried beans made with lard, served in a huge fried flour tortilla with copious quantities of processed cheese. (Can you say "serious bloating"?)

Everyone is a bit different. One person may classify a particular food as too tasty, while someone else may consider it just plain tasty, and therefore good. Have you ever noticed that certain foods seem tasty, whereas other, somewhat similar foods seem too tasty? What distinguishes them for you?

When you take a good look at the list above, the pattern is pretty clear: Foods that are too tasty aren't true to what you'd find in nature. They've been altered. They are synthetic products or whole foods with artificial ingredients added. As I mentioned earlier, many food companies manipulate foods in an attempt to give them that too-tasty appeal so that people will tend to overeat them. That means more profit for them—but more fat and disease for us. My recommendation? Focus on eating real foods and whole grains each day. You'll thank me in ten years. Or you could just keep hitting those 100-calorie packs. But if you do, my bet is that way before ten years from now you'll need bigger jeans—and you'll be considering membership in the powdered fiber flavor of the month club.

Chapter 6
Fat People Eat Calorie-Dense Foods

We may find in the long run that tinned food is a deadlier weapon than the machine-gun.

—George Orwell

Here's a salient factoid: a typical fast-food value meal has the same amount of calories as eighteen apples. Eighteen! I've seen buddies knock back two fast-food value meals while watching a football game on Sunday afternoon, but I haven't seen any of them go through 12 pounds of pippins by the fourth quarter.

What does this tell me? That Mother Nature has our back. She gave us real food—and because we evolved eating real food, it's what our bodies are best equipped to handle. As discussed in chapter 5, real food has so many benefits. Here are just a few that are relevant to this chapter:

- Real food usually provides a moderate amount of calories, naturally packaged with plenty of fiber to help you feel full and satisfied for longer.
- Real food controls your blood sugar and insulin levels so you can avoid energy swings and diabetes.
- Real food regulates your appetite (thanks to the previous two benefits) so you're less likely to overeat.
- Real food provides optimum nutrition to help you remain healthy for life.

This leads me to the topic of energy density, which is the amount of energy (calories) per unit of food. There are foods that don't take up much space but pack some serious energy (think sausage or brownies). There are also foods that take

As you can see, the caloric density of Tokyo is more than two dozen times that of the entire state of Wyoming.
TOKYO 12,790,000
WYOMING 493,782
BIZARROCOMIC.BLOGSPOT.COM
Dist. by King Features
PIRARO 10-18-10

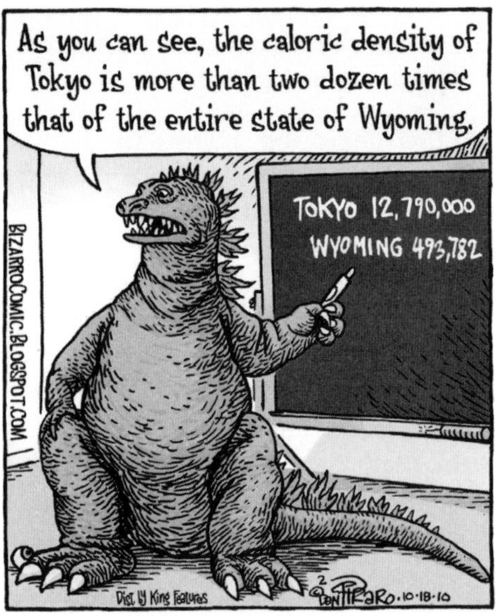

Bizarro, reprinted by permission of Dan Piraro.

up a lot of space but don't contain much energy (think lettuce or oranges). It's hard to rack up excess energy (calories) from most whole, real foods.

Understanding energy density (and applying that information) gives you much more control over one of the most important factors in winning the battle of the bulge: appetite. Most people feel as though they have no control over their appetite, so they try to ignore it (which doesn't seem to work in the long run) or look to supplements, drugs, or other artificial means to control it. Meanwhile, a much simpler and more healthful solution is available, based on one profound fact: Appetite isn't generally regulated by the number of calories you eat; it's mainly based on the volume of food you eat. Simply put, your appetite is based on the total volume of food (minus the air that gets pumped into processed foods, such as cakes, marshmallows, puffed cereals, and the like) that passes through your digestive tract. If you eat a high volume of food, you will feel satisfied. The less volume you eat, the hungrier you will feel.[1,2]

Caloric Density of Food

Calories per pound

Salad	100
Fruit	300
Potato	500
Rice	500
Beans	500
Ice Cream	1200
Bread	1500
Sugar	1800
CHOCOLATE	2500

Research also indicates that most people eat 3 to 5 pounds of food a day, and as we come close to taking in 4 pounds of food for the day, most of us feel satiated.[3] The thing is, this can be 4 pounds of celery, or it can be 4 pounds of candy bars. We tend to stop once we reach 3 to 5 pounds of food, regardless of what that food is or its calorie density.

Yet there are obviously some big differences in volume, energy density, and nutritional value between celery and candy bars, right? You bet, and here are some extreme examples to prove it. (Note that I'm showing calories only to help illustrate the point and address energy density. Don't get wrapped up in the exact numbers.)

- 4 pounds of raw veggies will provide about 400 calories (and lots of volume)
- 4 pounds of raw fruits will provide about 1,000 calories (and lots of volume)
- 4 pounds of cooked whole grains or legumes will provide about 1,600 calories (and some volume)

- 4 pounds of nuts or seeds will provide about 10,000 calories (and not much volume)
- 4 pounds of steak, bacon, toaster pastries, sugary cereals, or cheese will provide about 10,000 calories (and not much volume)

A Formula for Fatness

People who struggle with excess weight tend to fill up on calorie-dense processed foods. Remember, anytime you take in more energy (calories) than you're putting out, the energy will be stored (as fat) for your body to use at a later time. That's a formula for fatness. But if you eat 4 pounds of whole, real food with low calorie density overall, you'll get lots of nutrients, naturally packaged with an amount of calories that your body can handle.

Although I'm not a fan of calorie counting, I do recognize that calories and calorie density have a bearing on fitness, so let's take a closer look at the equation. First, here are the typical amounts of different foods that most people in the United States consume on an average day:[3]

Food	Quantity
Meat, dairy, or eggs	2 pounds
Fruits and vegetables	1 ½ pounds
Grains (usually refined)	½ pound
Sugars, fats, and oils	½ pound
Total quantity	4 ½ pounds
Calories per day	about 3,700

What if we switched this around? Here's my proposal:

Food	Quantity
Fruits and vegetables	2 ½ pounds
Whole grains and legumes	1 pound
Nuts and seeds	⅓ pound
Meat, dairy, or eggs	⅓ pound
Sugars, fats, and oils	1 to 2 ounces
Total quantity	4 ¼ pounds
Calories per day	about 2,075

If we prioritize and eat nutritious, real foods with fairly low calorie density, there isn't much room left for processed, calorie-dense foods. You have 3 to 5 pounds of food to work with each day. So think about it: What will your 4 pounds be?

Why Sweat the Small Stuff

Remember back in chapter 5, where I illustrated the difference between a fit person's diet and a fat person's diet using pie charts? Remember that bombshell that I dropped, saying that it doesn't matter whether that 15 percent slice of a fit person's diet is comprised of beans and other legumes or grass-fed beef, wild fish, free-range eggs, or dairy products? I lied. I believe it does matter. And as you can probably imagine, I think sticking with plant-based foods is your best bet.

It's not such a big deal, really. It boils down to swapping a minimal amount of meat, eggs, or dairy products for more peas and beans. To get down to specifics, it might mean replacing 8 ounces of grass-fed beef, 8 ounces of organic yogurt, and two eggs with 2 cups of cooked legumes.

But for some reason, contemplating this type of swap freaks people out. The top concern I hear is that substituting legumes for meat, eggs, and dairy will result in too many carbs, which most people associate with weight gain and increased body fat. Because anticarb sentiments have become so entrenched, let's step back and examine how this food swap actually works out (note that the values are approximate).

Type of Nutrient	Animal Products	Most Legumes	National Exchange
	8 ounces grass-fed beef, 1 cup 2 percent Greek yogurt, and 2 free-range eggs	2 cups cooked beans or peas	
Calories	770	400	330 fewer calories
Fat (grams)	38	2	36 fewer grams of fat
Carbohydrates (grams)	11	79	68 more grams of carbohydrate
Fiber (grams)	0	31	31 more grams of fiber
Protein (grams)	92	32	60 fewer grams of protein

All of these numbers are interesting, but two really catch my eye: 31 more grams of fiber and 330 fewer calories. What those numbers tell me is that this dietary swap will lead to more regular bowel movements and less body fat.

The carbs in beans and peas contain a lot of resistant starch and fiber.[4] These forms of carbohydrate pass through the digestive tract without being absorbed and help you feel more full for a longer time after meals. They also help control blood sugar levels, which could help control cravings. And even though I'm not big on calorie counting, it's obvious that eating 330 fewer calories daily is a substantial decrease, and if you eat this way regularly, you will see a reduction in your waistline—and maybe even your bottom line, if you get my drift.

Chapter 7
Fat People Eat Mostly Animal Proteins

I am oppressed with a dread of living forever. That is the only disadvantage of vegetarianism.

—George Bernard Shaw

Oh good, you're still here. I thought you might bail on me after reading the chapter title. Remember what I said back in chapter 5, about how it doesn't matter whether that 15 percent slice of a fit person's diet is comprised of beans and other legumes or grass-fed beef, wild fish, free-range eggs, or dairy products—and how at the end of chapter 6 I said that this was actually a lie? (I certainly hope you remember this, since it was the topic of discussion at the end of the previous chapter!) I've decided that the brief discussion of why sweat the small stuff at the end of the previous chapter just won't do it. In fact, I've decided to devote an entire chapter to the topic of plant-based protein.

Why? Because Americans are fat, and our confusion about protein isn't helping. In a 2010 survey, participants were asked to identify statements they believed to be accurate about dietary protein. A whopping 72 percent of respondents didn't know that plant-based foods contain protein.[1] Yikes! The survey also revealed that 49 percent of Americans are trying to consume more protein. The theme to *Jaws* might be appropriate here (hmm, or maybe *Titanic*). Somehow, I get the feeling that bacon and sausage will be the way Americans try to bump up protein intake.

Still, it should come as no surprise that most Americans lack information about protein from plant sources. After all, the nation tends to get its nutritional advice from TV commercials, and there are entire ad campaigns dedicated to the "benefits" of meat, dairy, and eggs. But when's the last time you saw a riveting TV commercial pushing dried beans and peas and extolling their protein content? The popular media isn't doing folks a lot of favors on this front either. If you ask John Q. Public about the merits of a plant-based diet, you're likely to hear that he's concerned about two things: eating too many carbs and getting fat, and not getting enough protein and losing muscle as a result.

Time for some nutrition triage. My first order of business is to assure John Q. Public that eating plenty of whole, unprocessed plant-based foods doesn't make people overweight. If you doubt this, go find all the people you know who have forty-two-inch waists and high blood pressure from eating too much quinoa, lentils, pears, and collard greens. I'll wait. (Good thing I've been meaning to read *War and Peace*, and that I happen to have a copy of it handy.)

Food for Thought

Do you doubt that plant-based foods are a good source of protein? Excellent! Let's play a fun little game.

Consider a typical fast-food burger versus steamed asparagus. As a percentage of total calories, which has more protein? If you chose the hamburger, you're wrong. It only has about 18 percent protein, whereas asparagus has 34 percent.

Now you're probably wondering if asparagus is a freak of the vegetable world, so let's play again. Consider a hardboiled egg versus grilled tofu. As a percentage of total calories, which has more protein? If you chose the egg, you're wrong. It has about 33 percent protein, whereas tofu has 40 percent.

But rather than continuing to play this somewhat silly little game, let's cut to the chase. Take a few minutes to read through the following table, which lists the percentage of calories from protein in various healthful plant-based foods. And for comparison, another table follows showing a few foods that fall into the categories of junk food or foods from animal sources.[2] For context, you should know that values below 12 percent represent a relatively low percentage of protein, values between 12 and 20 are moderate, and values greater than 20 are high. Also note that just because a food comes in at below 20 percent doesn't make it bad in any way; it just indicates that it might be a good idea to consume other foods with a higher protein content to round out your nutrition.

Plant-based food	Percentage of calories from protein
Vegetables	
Spinach	39%
Asparagus	34%
Broccoli	27%
Squash	24%
Sea vegetables	20%

Plant-based food	Percentage of calories from protein
Grains	
Hempseed bread	30%
Sprouted-grain bread	20%
Oats	17%
Amaranth	16%
Quinoa	14%
Legumes	
Veggie burgers made with soy	50%
Tofu	40%
Tempeh	34%
Edamame	30%
Lentils	30%
Peas	26%
Refried beans	24%
Hummus	18%
Nuts and Seeds	
Hempseeds	27%
Pumpkin seeds	23%
Flaxseeds	17%
Peanut butter	15%
Almonds	14%
Walnuts	14%
Miscellaneous	
Soy protein powder	80% to 85%
Pea protein powder	80%
Seitan (wheat gluten)	77%
Rice protein powder	75% to 80%
Hempseed protein powder	50% to 70%

Plant-based food	Percentage of calories from protein
Beverages	
Soymilk	30%
Hempseed milk	18%

And now for a point of comparison:

Animal-based food, refined food, and junk food	Percentage of calories from protein
Ground beef	45%
Salmon	44%
Eggs (whole)	33%
Cheese	33%
Cow's milk (2% fat)	27%
White bread	11%
White rice	9%
Ice cream	7%
Human breast milk	6%
Doughnuts	4%
Licorice	3%
Jam	0%

As the first table illustrates, the percentage of protein in many plant-based foods is balanced. So why are they typically regarded as poor sources of protein? The confusion probably has to do with a focus on grams of protein, rather than percentages. Although asparagus checks in at 34 percent protein, you'd have to eat two cups to get just 9 grams of protein. But look at the flip side. That's 9 grams of protein packaged together with only 80 total calories. This might be very bad news—if your goal of keeping up with the Joneses includes accruing ever more body fat. But if you're trying to achieve and maintain a lean body, then it's excellent news indeed.

How Much Is Enough?

I'd like to believe that I've convinced you at this point, but I know how much hysteria there is about getting enough protein, so let's do some math. Ideal protein intake ranges from 0.36 grams to 0.64 grams of protein per pound of body weight, depending on activity level.[3] So a 150-pound adult who plays video games in the basement all day should aim for about 54 grams of protein per day. Can our gamer easily get that much protein while parked in front of a video screen? Let's see:

Food	Protein (grams)
1 cup of cooked lentils with 2 tablespoons of ground hempseeds	29
2 slices of sprouted-grain bread with 2 tablespoons of peanut butter	16
1 cup of cooked brussels sprouts with ½ cup of cooked quinoa	9
Total	54

Folks, we have a winner! And given that our gamer probably doesn't devote a lot of attention to savoring meals, why not replace pizza, cookies, ice cream, and soda with fare that's a little more healthful. If nothing else, this person might burn a few more calories in the process of chewing and digesting whole plant foods.

For a 150 pound adult who lifts, runs, jumps, walks, bicycles, does yoga, and has a goal of keeping a lean and muscular body, consuming a bit more protein—up to 96 grams—is probably a smart idea.[4–7] At the end of this chapter, I'll outline a sample menu plan with even more protein packed in, to show you just how easy achieving that goal can be.

Variety Is the Spice of Life

I can almost hear what you're thinking: "But Ryan, if someone is eating like this, don't they need to make sure beans are consumed within twenty-seven minutes of grains—and only after reciting the Alarte Ascendare spell from Harry Potter?" Nope, introduce yourself to one of the biggest nutrition myths of all. For some reason, most people believe that plants don't contain all of the essential amino acids. This isn't accurate. Plant-based foods contain all of the essential amino acids in varying proportions.[8, 9] There's no need to do elaborate food combining to ensure you get the correct proportions of amino acids. As long as you consume a wide variety of plant-based foods and don't get stuck in a rut with certain foods for days on end, you'll get sufficient quantities of all of the essential amino acids, with nary a speck of animal protein in sight. Honestly, your body can't tell any difference between an amino acid from eggs and that same amino acid from lentils.

I feel so strongly about this that I'm willing to go out on what may seem like a limb (trust me, it's not). Here's the plain and simple truth: It's impossible to create a 100 percent plant-based diet that is deficient in protein as long as you meet the following four requirements:

1. **Eat enough energy (calories) to sustain a lean body.** When you eat enough to meet your energy needs, protein is free to play the roles it's supposed to in the body, like sustaining muscle mass and hormone levels. If you don't eat enough each day, the protein you consume may be diverted to other functions in the body, like producing energy. (This means you can wave good-bye to muscle mass, if you can lift your limp, withered arm to do that.)
2. **Don't overemphasize cereals, grains, and processed foods.** Don't go all North American and eat cereal for breakfast, a massive hoagie for lunch, pretzels for snacks, and pasta for dinner. This way of eating actually *is* too heavy in grains and low in protein, and this can lead to excess body fat. Fortunately, it's easy to up the protein density while sticking with plant-based foods; for example, you might try a green smoothie for breakfast, lentil and quinoa salad for lunch, fruits and nuts for snacks, or a tempeh burger for dinner.
3. **Don't go gorilla and only eat fruit.** Eating only fruit for a day or two is fine for recalibrating your appetite, cleansing your body, and clearing your head, but eating only fruit for an extended period of time can lead to amino acid deficiencies (and fatty acid deficiencies). In time, this means less muscle and ultimately a lower metabolism, making it harder to stay lean.
4. **Include at least ½ cup of beans or other legumes each day.** Eating closer to 1 cup of legumes daily would actually be ideal. Legumes are a rich source of lysine, the amino acid that tends to be deficient in most other plant-based foods, and grains in particular.[10–12] Unfortunately, this is where many people fall short. Often they don't eat many beans because of bloating and gas. There are solutions. Make sure you cook beans sufficiently and then chew them well. If this doesn't solve the problem, experiment with different varieties of beans and peas. You're likely to find some you tolerate well, especially smaller beans like lentils and split peas.

To build a house you need a certain amount of lumber, bricks, drywall, and nails. To build a fit body, you need a certain amount of each essential amino acid. Think of lysine as nails. It's great to have enough lumber, bricks, and drywall, but without enough nails (lysine), the house will fall apart. The average 150-pound adult needs about 2 to 3 grams of lysine per day.[5,11] To help you make sure you're getting enough, here's a list of the lysine content in some common plant-based foods:

Food	Lysine (grams)
Tofu, 1 cup cooked	2.2
Tempeh, 1 cup cooked	1.5
Lentils, 1 cup cooked	1.2
Split peas, 1 cup cooked	1.2
Chickpeas, 1 cup cooked	1.0
Cashew butter, ¼ cup	0.6
Pistachios, ⅓ cup	0.5
Quinoa, 1 cup cooked	0.4
Peanuts, ¼ cup	0.4
Almond butter, ¼ cup	0.4
Peanut butter, ¼ cup	0.4
Hempseeds, ¼ cup	0.4
Rolled oats, 1 cup cooked	0.3
Buckwheat, 1 cup cooked	0.3
Sunflower seed butter, ¼ cup	0.3
Brown rice, 1 cup cooked	0.2
Pearl barley, 1 cup cooked	0.1
Whole wheat bread, 2 slices	0.1

So, for our hypothetical 150-pound adult, eating 1 cup each of cooked lentils and quinoa and ⅓ cup of pistachios would provide enough lysine for the day. You might be tempted to think that lysine supplements are the easy way out, but I don't recommend them. They can be toxic to the kidneys in high amounts. Plus, supplementing with single amino acids can create other amino acid imbalances.

Dishing It Up

As you've probably noticed by now, I'm not big on giving specific dietary recommendations. But people tend to get pretty worked up about the protein issue, so I thought I'd include a sample menu showing how easy it is to get enough protein from plant-based foods. The following day of meals would provide an ideal amount of protein for someone who is physically active and weighs between 165 and 185 pounds (and way more protein than our 150-pound basement gamer requires). If you weigh less than 165 pounds or more than 185 pounds or have a different activity level, you'd simply adjust the amounts accordingly.

Breakfast Shake (process in a blender until smooth)
Almond milk (1 cup)
Frozen fruit (½ cup)
Kale (3 large leaves)
Hempseeds (2 tablespoons)
Ground flaxseeds (1 tablespoon)

Lunch
Green beans (1 cup, steamed)
Lentils (1 cup cooked)
Amaranth (½ cup cooked)
Pistachios (¼ cup)

Afternoon Snack
Roasted chickpeas (⅓ cup)
Pumpkin seeds (2 tablespoons)
Raw veggies or fresh fruit

Dinner
Portobello mushrooms (2 large, grilled)
Cauliflower (1 to 2 cups, steamed)
Sweet potato, baked (fist-sized)
Salad greens with ground hempseeds and tahini dressing
Tofu or tempeh (2 ounces)

Just one caveat about eating this way: You do need to take a vitamin B_{12} supplement, and depending on your overall dietary patterns, other supplements may be warranted. Also feel free to use a protein supplement, especially if it will help you sleep better at night (more on that topic in chapter 13). There are plenty of plant-based protein powders available, made from peas, rice, hempseeds, or other ingredients.

One final note to set your mind at ease: Protein requirements are estimated based on metabolic needs over time. While this is often stated in terms of daily intake, this doesn't mean that you must consume this exact amount every day. Rather, you just need to consume this much protein on an average basis over the course of several days.

Got Motivation?

Still wondering if plant-based eating is for you? I'm sure you've heard all kinds of arguments in favor of it. Clearly those haven't fully swayed you. So I'll just leave you with this thought: In the United States, we kill and eat almost 17,000 animals per minute, or about 1 million animals per hour. Folks, the population of Dallas, Texas, is 1.2 million people. Over the course of a lifetime, the average American omnivore will eat about 21,000 animals.[13] That's akin to eating the entire population of Laguna Beach, California. I'm just sayin'.

Chapter 8
Fat People Drink Calories

I think all addiction starts with soda. Every junkie did soda first. But no one counts that. Maybe they should. The soda connection is clear. Why isn't a presidential commission looking into this?

—Chris Rock

Energy drinks, juice, milk, and soda—and maybe some beer, wine, or other alcoholic beverages. Sound tasty? Check! Big contributor to fatness? Double-check! High-calorie beverages (including some you might think of as healthful, such as flavored nondairy milk and fruit juice) are typically recommended for two types of people: sumo wrestlers and those going into hibernation. So if storing body fat is a high priority, then liquid calories are your best friend.

How Sweet It Isn't

Why are high-calorie drinks, especially the sugary kind, so fat promoting? For starters, despite containing lots of calories, they don't do much to make you feel full. So even after drinking 500 calories (for example, two 20-ounce soft drinks or three 12-ounce beers), you'll still be hungry. That wouldn't be the case if you ate 500 calories worth of cooked brown rice or lentils (about 2½ cups) or steamed broccoli (about 10 cups!).

And remember, kids – not only is milk a fattening health hazard, but when you're drinking milk, it means a sad & lonely calf somewhere isn't!
Aa Bb Cc
2+2=4
BK
BIZARRO.COM
BUZZKILL the LUNCHLADY
©DAN PIRARO
1·25·06

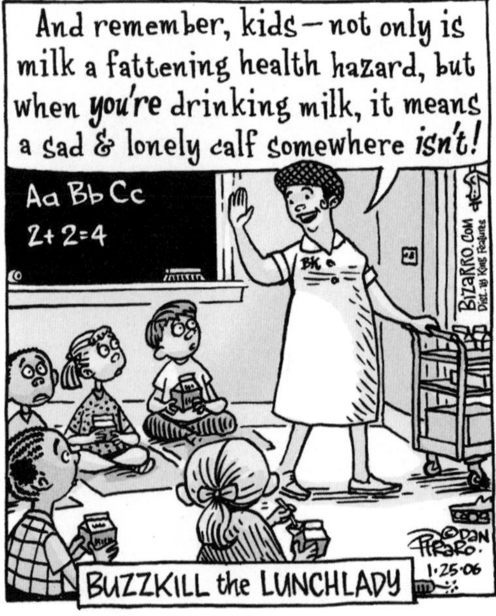

Bizarro, reprinted by permission of Dan Piraro.

Another problem is that sugary drinks cause a rapid spike in blood sugar, resulting in increased output of insulin to manage all of that sugar. High insulin levels promote body fat in two ways: by turning off metabolism of stored fat for energy and by storing the excess blood sugar. Initially, the excess sugars are stored in the muscles and liver in a complex, starchlike molecule known as glycogen. But if blood sugar remains elevated (which it will if you sip on sugary beverages throughout the day), the sugars will be converted into new fat and stored in adipose tissue (fat), typically on the belly, hips, thighs, and buttocks—not a pretty picture.

The Fruit, the Whole Fruit, and Nothing but the Fruit

A lot of people have a hard time believing that 100 percent natural fruit juice can be less than healthful. But consider this: a single glass of fruit juice contains all of the sugars from several pieces of fruit—sans the fiber, which promotes feelings of fullness and slows the release of the sugars from fruit into the bloodstream. Calories in one orange? 62. Calories in 8 ounces of orange juice? 110. Fiber in one orange? 3 grams. Fiber in 8 ounces of orange juice? Zip, zero, zilch, nada. You do the math.

Sure, if you're an athlete with a demanding training regimen or are ill and having a hard time with solid foods, high-calorie beverages may be helpful. But assuming that you don't fall into either of those categories, consuming these beverages regularly can, and probably will, lead to fat gain. Still, if you choose to keep drinking sugary beverages, at least you won't have to feel alone. Soft drinks account for 47 percent of the added sugars in the typical U.S. diet,[1] making them the primary source of added sugars for many Americans. So what's wrong with being normal? First, take a look around you and see if you really want to look like the average American. And second, if you're consuming more than 100 calories (25 grams) of added sugars per day, I hate to break it to you, but your diet sucks—probably on a jumbo soft drink.

Downsides of Diet Beverages

But what about diet and light beverages? Ah yes, good old artificial sweeteners; they're fairly popular too. In 2008, 65 percent of American households bought at least one product with an artificial sweetener.[2] And between 1989 and 2004, the amount of artificial sweeteners ingested from beverages increased by 38 percent.[3] While some people are successful in utilizing diet beverages to help control weight, for many people these beverages cause rebound sugar cravings.[2, 3] In fact, some studies have shown that increased use of artificial sweeteners is associated with weight gain.[2, 4] The reasons for this aren't yet known, but it may involve something that's very difficult to change: how the human brain is wired. Researchers believe that using artificial sweeteners may support a habit of preferring a sweet taste. Yet because the body doesn't obtain the calories it expects in association with that flavor, appetite is actually increased. Another bummer is that diet beverages raise your "sweet threshold," meaning your taste buds get jaded. If you doubt this, try eating a few blueberries after drinking a 12-ounce diet soda. The blueberries won't taste very sweet.

Booze

Don't fool yourself into thinking that alcohol doesn't count here. If you don't drink already, the benefits of drinking fewer calories gives you another good reason not to start. If you do drink, be aware that alcohol consumption above one to two drinks per day can displace nutrients and increase health risks.[5, 6] Oh, and you'll also exponentially increase your chances of falling off a balcony—or just acting like an ass.

As if you need further reason to avoid alcohol, consider this: As with excessive sugar intake, alcohol can suppress the body's fat metabolism. Worse yet, it causes the excess, nonmetabolized fat to be deposited in the abdominal area.[7] Aside from this not being a good look for hitting the beach, carrying excess abdominal fat is associated with increased risk for a wide range of health conditions, including heart disease, high blood pressure, stroke, type 2 diabetes, and some types of cancer. That's *really* not a pretty picture.

Sipping for Success

So, what should you drink? My advice is to mostly stick to water and tea (such as herbal, rooibos, green, white, black, or oolong). These have been shown to help keep people lean and healthy. For a refreshing and cleansing start to your day, try a glass of cold water with a squeeze of fresh lemon or lime juice. Save caloric beverages for special occasions or forgo them completely. As for diet beverages, just forget they even exist.

As with all areas of nutrition, set yourself up for success with beverage intake. Don't try to completely avoid beverages you really love; instead, aim to drink them in moderation—extreme moderation (now there's an oxymoron for you). If you're really attached to a small glass of 100 percent juice in the morning or almond milk in a breakfast shake, or maybe even the occasional beer or glass of wine, don't deprive yourself—though you might want to dilute that fruit juice with water. You need to find a strategy that will work for you in the long run. But if you keep on slamming down mugs of soda, juice, or chocolate soymilk and the reflection you see in the mirror is reminiscent of Santa Claus, don't say I didn't warn you.

Chapter 9
Fat People Eat Fast Food

There are many of us who cannot but feel dismal about the future of various cultures. Often it is hard not to agree that we are becoming culinary nitwits, dependent upon fast foods and mass kitchens and megavitamins for our basically rotten nourishment.

—M. F. K. Fisher

Want to know my biggest turnoff, hands down? When I see a girl pull up to a fast-food drive-through window. But if I see a girl loading up on kale and lentils from a salad bar, that's a big turn-on. If she chases the kale with green tea, I'd consider proposing on the spot.

Since I'm being honest here, people who eat fast food give me the heebie-jeebies. I'm sure you've read some of those headlines about bizarre crimes at fast-food joints ("Man Holds Up Jack in the Box, Comes Back for Lunch" and "Man Robs Arby's with Samurai Sword," to quote a couple). They seem sort of funny . . . until you realize that the humorous stories are just the tip of the iceberg, and that drive-through workers actually do get physically assaulted by people who are more than a little disappointed about some aspect of the "food" or "service" tendered ("McNuggets Rage Sends Woman into Drive-Thru Frenzy" and "Taco Bell Burrito Price Hike Leads to Texas Shootout," to quote a couple more). These kinds of stories make fast-food fanatics seem like people scoring drugs (hmm, "Drunk Pregnant Woman Tries to Rob Taco Joint," for drug money, I kid you not).

Nevertheless, some folks believe that fast food isn't addictive. Sure . . . and I'm the father of three elves named Fernando, Kuwalski, and Bergomand. I don't see people ready to pull out an épée at the farmers' market when zucchini is out of season.

Fast-Food Nation

You know it. I know it. The drive-through clerk at the twenty-four-hour fast-food joint knows it. People still eat fast food—a lot of it. Yet we all know that fast food is a suboptimal source of nutrition. So who's actually eating it? Well, about fifty-four million customers are served by McDonald's each day.[1] And that's just McDonald's. Folks, that's the population of Pennsylvania, New Jersey, New

York, Connecticut, Rhode Island, Massachusetts, New Hampshire, Vermont, and Maine—combined. That means more than one-fifth of the U.S. population is served by McDonald's each day.

Americans spend about 10 percent of their disposable income on food. In the 1930s, Americans spent 30 percent of their disposable income on food.[2] Plus, nearly half of every food dollar in the United States is spent outside the home.[3] Americans now spend more money on fast food than they spend on books, magazines, movies, music, and newspapers combined. Here's an idea: eating out less often—and particularly eating fast food less often—could make for a leaner body. The side effects are awesome too: improved health, fewer carbon emissions, less fast-food packaging strewn across the landscape, and the list goes on.

The Whys Have It

Okay, so we know that millions of people eat fast food each day. Here's the big question: Why? Fortunately, we have a study titled "Why Eat at Fast-Food Restaurants: Reported Reasons among Frequent Customers" to give us some answers.[4] By the way, upon reading this title, I felt like it was Christmas morning. I couldn't wait to see what fast-food peeps revealed as their top reasons for eating substances that barely qualify as food. So with no further ado, here are the most frequently reported reasons for eating at fast-food restaurants:

- It's quick.
- It's easy to get.
- It tastes good.

And here are some of the least frequently reported reasons for eating at fast-food restaurants:

- It's a way of socializing with family and friends.
- It's nutritious.
- It's fun and entertaining.

Amusing answers, right? I wonder if fast-food fans think the top three reasons healthy people eat nutritious foods look something like this:

- It takes a long time.
- It's a pain in the ass.
- It's bland and unappetizing.

Sure, sometimes healthful living is complicated, time-consuming, tedious, and built upon denial of life's pleasures—but usually because people approach it thinking it has to be that way. Although staying fit and healthy does require a consistent and intentional approach, the idea that it has to be difficult is a self-imposed obstacle. Really, how hard is it to eat delicious, healthful food and do energizing workouts—especially when doing so makes you feel excellent day in, day out? There's no universal law decreeing that health-supporting habits have to be onerous. Choose an approach that works for you.

And now, back to our regularly scheduled programming: the aforementioned study "Why Eat at Fast-Food Restaurants: Reported Reasons among Frequent Customers." The results of that study leave me dumbfounded yet optimistic—and also a little sad. Let's deal with "dumbfounded" first. Did you notice that "It's nutritious" is near the bottom of the list of reasons why people eat fast food? Apparently people *know* that fast food doesn't promote health, but they still choose to eat it on a regular basis. This supports my theory that knowledge isn't the limiting factor behind poor nutrition in America.

Still, the top three reasons for eating fast food give good cause for optimism. If people are eating fast food because it's quick, easy, and tastes good, all of those qualifiers could also apply to more healthful fast-food options. But more than anything, this study makes me feel a little sad. It illustrates the power of both advertising and social norms. Children in the United States view up to forty thousand commercials each year, and advertisers spend more than $2.5 billion per year to promote restaurants.[5] "But Ryan," you say, "$2.5 billion isn't that much." Don't tell that to the folks behind the Five-A-Day campaign to increase fruit and vegetable consumption (now "Fruits and Veggies—More Matters"). They were spending about $9.5 *million* each year.[6] Break out your abacus. This means restaurant advertisers were spending about 260 times more than the Five-A-Day campaign. Heck, the advertising budget for one popular candy bar is eight times larger than that of the Five-A-Day campaign.

I think people eat fast food because they don't consider other options—and may not even be aware of other options. They grow up seeing commercials for fast food, their parents eat it, their friends eat it, their coworkers eat it, and so on. Eating fast food is just what people do in America. My guess is that most of these people haven't experienced many other food options, and that's a shame.

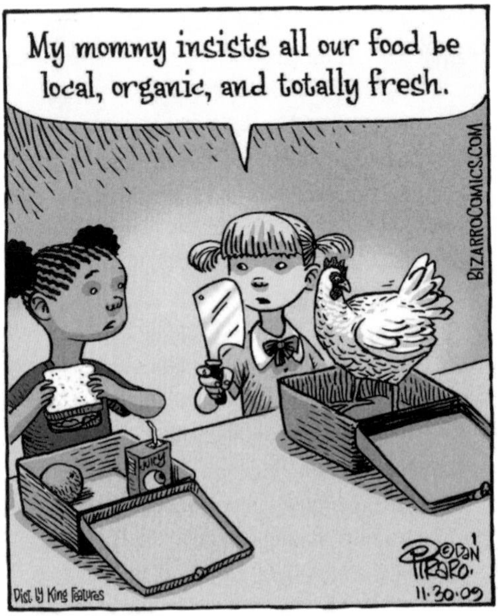

Bizarro, reprinted by permission of Dan Piraro.

The Fast-Food Fix

The fact is, taking thirty minutes to prepare food or stopping at a grocery store to gather your daily bounty is also quick and easy, and the results can be very tasty. So, what's really driving the fast-food phenomenon? Is there something deeper? Honestly, I think reasons like quick, easy, and tasty are just a way to rationalize an addiction to fast food. Yes, I said "addiction." People who frequent these places aren't usually opting for the green salads or fruit bowls; they're eating for a fix—often in an effort to add some stimulation to their lives.

And then there's that wretched excuse that this way of eating is "cheap." That's just an illusion. As Michael Pollan, author, activist, and professor of journalism at the University of California, Berkeley, says in the food film *Fresh*, "There's no such thing as cheap food. The real cost of the food is paid somewhere." If you aren't willing to fork out at the cash register, rest assured that the true cost will be charged to the environment, your health, or the public purse in the form of subsidies.

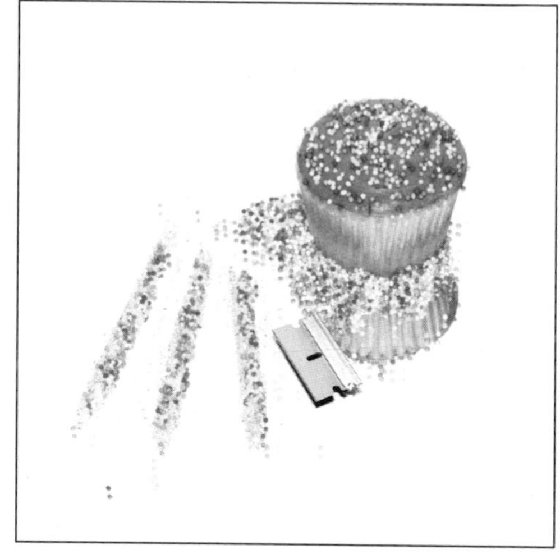

Thanks to Jon Raine (jonphotography.com) for this image.

Here's an idea: You know how we don't have crack houses on every corner, and how heroin purveyors aren't allowed to advertise on TV—or offer a free theme toy with every dime bag? How about getting standard fast food off the streets or completely revamping the food these places offer? If fast-food crack, er, crap isn't available, people won't be able to develop an addiction to it.

But until the day when addictive fast foods are banned, be wary—be very wary—of fast-food advertising claims. They have sneaky ways of making you think their food is a nutritious option. You may have heard some of these prestidigitations (for you nonliterary types, that means hocus-pocus). One fast-food chain actually claims their offerings are "way better than fast food." What? Isn't that sort of like saying, "It's way better than crack; it's cocaine."

Warning: Rant ahead. You know how I just said one potential solution is to revamp the menus at fast-food joints? Countless food companies are making considerable efforts to do just that—and not just fast-food chains, but also purveyors of packaged goods. In 2008, a Grocery Manufacturers Association's poll revealed that 92 percent of companies said they were reformulating existing products or introducing new products to have reduced fat or sugar.[7]

La-de-frickin'-da. As you'll recall from chapter 5, I believe that processed foods shouldn't exist in the first place. I don't want a sugar-free sandwich pseudocookie. I don't want a dusting of whole grains on a toaster pastry.

And I definitely don't want a lower-sodium dead-animal sandwich from a fast-food joint. We don't need more processed foods. They generally aren't health promoting, and they never will be. We need more real food and more community involvement in food production.

Easy but Not Cheap

Let's take a minute to revisit the idea that one merit of fast food is that it's cheap. After all, one fast-food chain even claims that if you just buy items from their value menu, you'll see a great return on your investment in these challenging economic times. Excellent! Um, if by "great return on investment" they mean these kinds of long-term outcomes:

- Monthly prescription bills around $200 for blood pressure, cholesterol, and diabetes medications
- A cardiac bypass operation for $100,000
- Nonsustainable foods that contribute to deterioration of the planet
- The suffering and eventual slaughter of countless animals
- Low-paying jobs for people working at every level of the fast-food supply line, from field and feedlot to drive-through window
- An inability to regulate fullness cues while eating, and never feeling quite satisfied
- Lots of new pants once the forty-inch (and beyond) waist is attained

Heart attack with extra cheese, heart attack with bacon, double bypass no pickles, --hey! Where's my diabetes and large stroke?
RATION
RECEPTION
DAN PIRARO 9-27-06
Dist. by King Features BIZARRO.COM

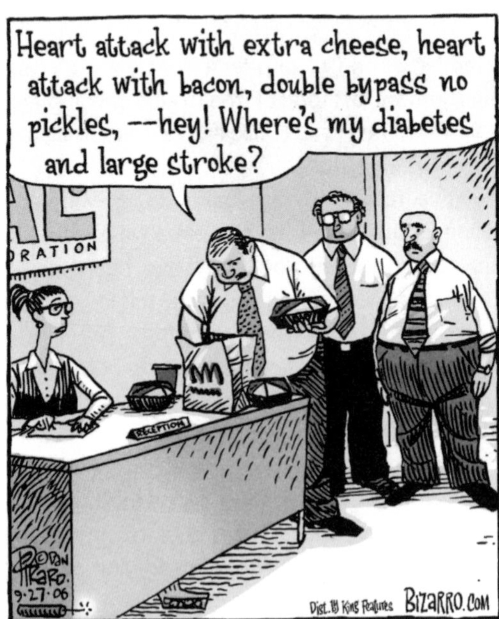

Bizarro, reprinted by permission of Dan Piraro.

The fact is, to save money in tough economic times many people do switch from midtier restaurants to lower-priced fast-food chains. As you can imagine, I think that's lame. I'd offer my own explanation why, but I don't think anything I say can top this statistic from *Freakonomics: A Rogue Economist Explores the Hidden Side of Everything*, by Steven Levitt and Stephen Dubner: "Economist Kevin Murphy found that a cheeseburger costs $2.50 more than a salad in long-term health implications."[8]

So, is fast food really saving you money?

Exploding Livers

As this chapter draws to a close, I'd like to leave you with some food for thought. Actually, it's a recipe—a recipe for disaster: Combining even a brief flirtation with fast food with too little exercise can induce rapid and profound elevations in liver enzymes and liver fat. At least that's what one small study found.[9] Among healthy volunteers who took a "fast-food challenge" for four weeks, sharp increases in the liver enzyme alanine transaminase occurred after just one week, and levels quadrupled over the study period. Why should you care? When this happens, it's a good indication your liver—your body's hardworking organ of detoxification—is inflamed and damaged. Another bummer is that just one fatty meal like those served in fast-food joints not only hurts your liver, but it also plays havoc with your blood vessels.[10]

But do we really need rigorous, double-blind scientific studies to tell us that fast food isn't good for us? You can conduct your own study right now. Walk to a local fast-food restaurant and take a good, long look at the people eating there. Do you really want to look or feel like most of those people?

Chapter 10
Fat People Don't Have Basic Food-Preparation Skills

Cooking is one of the oldest arts and one which has rendered us the most important service in civic life.

—Jean-Anthelme Brillat-Savarin

If your proudest food-prep achievement is memorizing the microwave cooking time for pizza rolls, well, how can I put this diplomatically? You won't be earning any gold stars from me. Sorry. And in case you had any doubt, I also don't count a doughnut run, tipping the delivery guy, or making boxed macaroni and cheese as food-preparation skills.

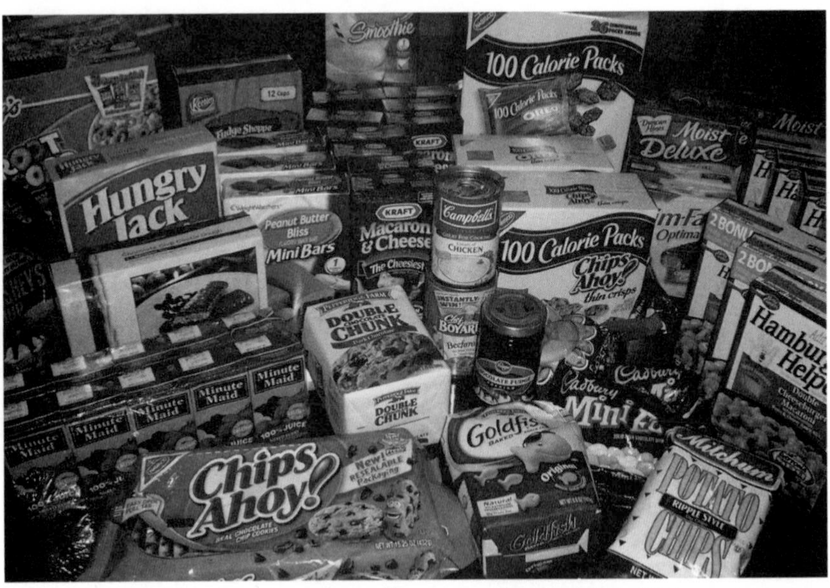

This is what one of my clients cleaned out of her cupboards after doing a kitchen makeover.

To earn your cooking merit badge—and to start shedding some pounds—you're going to need to know how to steam broccoli, cook rice, chop pineapple, and boil lentils. Yes, you're going to need to use a knife, cutting board, measuring cups, saucepans, and maybe even a stove.

They Like to Watch

Most Americans are pretty good at shopping (including at the grocery store) and eating. The limiting factor lies in between: basic food prep. When fat people walk through the produce section, they turn a blind eye to the kale, chard, beets, and mangoes because they don't know what to do with them. Eventually they end up in the snack foods aisles, where they stock up on chips, cookies, and snack cakes. And then they wonder why their pants don't fit.

The fact is, despite the immense popularity of television cooking shows, American adults spend only about thirty minutes per day on food prep and clean-up.[1] That number is impressive . . . for a six-year-old, but not for a healthy, fit adult. What are people doing with the rest of their discretionary time? Well, statistics show that they're busy with three plus hours of TV and almost two hours sitting behind the wheel of a car.[1,2] Let's face it: some folks care more about watching *Iron Chef* than they do about their health—or about doing their own cooking!

Give Mom a Little Respect

As many times as I've prepared my own meals, something always strikes me as I admire the finished product: I have more respect for the food. When I take the time and effort to cook healthful foods, I'm less likely to double up on portions or mindlessly eat while reading the latest issue of *People Magazi* . . . er . . . *Men's Fitness*. And on the rare occasions when I make cookies or other treats, I portion them out rather than eating most of the batch in one sitting.

Today, so many people lack appreciation for the food they eat. It's easy to slam down mass-produced foods without a second thought. Not only are they typically *too tasty*, you also don't have to expend much effort to obtain them. But what if you spent an hour of thought, time, and energy devising a menu, then buying and prepping ingredients and cooking your meal? You'd probably be more likely to savor each bite—allowing your brain to get the message that your stomach is full so that you don't eat a day's worth of food in one sitting. To take this attitude of gratitude to an entirely new level, you might even consider actually

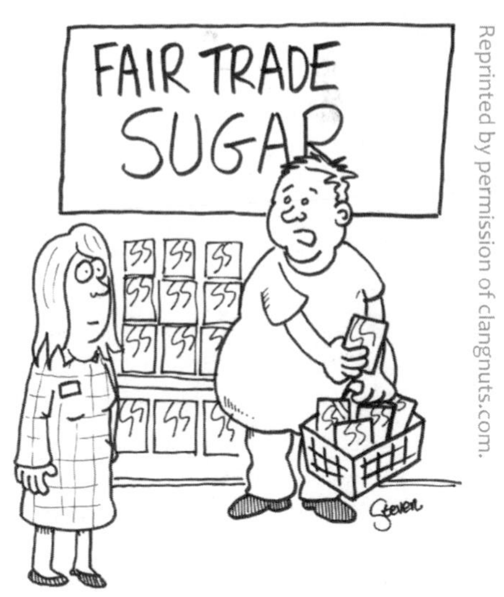

"I'm just doing my bit to help all the poor farmers in Belize"

growing some of your food. Talk about respect—when I grow an heirloom tomato, I treat it like a family treasure—up to the point where I gratefully devour it!

Sadly, the days of homegrown food seem to be long gone. Heck, for most people even local food is a stretch. The demand for packaged and exotic foods is out of control. In the United States, the average food item travels 1,020 miles before it reaches the dinner table.[3] (As though Americans actually sit down at the table to eat.) If it weren't for fossil fuels, we wouldn't be able to stock our pantries with all of those chips, cookies, and snack cakes—or run our freezers to store all of those microwave meals. And although a microwave dinner may seem appealing because it takes only a few minutes to prepare, remember that it took Mother Nature thousands of years to produce the oil for the plastic wrapper and at least a few decades to grow the trees for the cardboard tray. Don't piss her off.

The Carbon Hoofprint

Now that you know that most of us rely on food produced hundreds, if not thousands, of miles away, you're probably thinking that the pace of global climate change is going to snowball. (So long, Florida!) To keep things in perspective, bear in mind that while eating local is great on many levels, transportation miles are responsible for only 11 percent of the greenhouse gas emissions attributable to food. The remainder of those emissions are created during food production, particularly raising cattle.

As far as carbon footprint is concerned, eating a vegan diet one day per week achieves a greater greenhouse gas reduction than buying only locally sourced food.[3] Additionally, if the world's growing population decided to eat the same amount of meat that the world's affluent now consume, we would need 67 percent more land than the earth has.[4]

Food-Preparation Options

Preparing food can be simple; there's no need for marathon kitchen sessions. Don't believe me? Consider raw foodists, who don't eat anything cooked to a temperature much above one hundred degrees Fahrenheit. They tend to be healthier than most of the people who eat cooked food, so becoming best buddies with your stove and oven is entirely optional.

The advertisements of most food manufacturers will try to convince you that preparing meals from scratch is too difficult. Ignore them. In North America you can walk into almost any supermarket and purchase nearly any food you want. Even if you've convinced yourself that you're just "too busy" to spend much time on food prep, you'll find that most supermarkets offer precut veggies and fruits and other healthful whole foods that require little to no cooking time. How much easier can it get?

Sometimes getting started is the hardest part, so even though I encourage you to cook from scratch, don't feel that you have to reinvent the wheel each time you do so. To make your life easier, I recommend that you develop some food-preparation rituals. These rituals don't involve mantras and Ouija boards (unless you want them to), and they definitely don't involve eye of newt or anything similarly unsavory. What they do involve is creating a routine and making it a part of your day or week. Here are a few options for you to explore:

Option 1: Weekly rituals. Set aside a few hours one day per week to plan your menus for that week, and then shop and prepare as much food in advance as you can. This investment of time will pay off during the rest of the week, when you'll have only minimal prep and cooking to do. Plus, imagine how great it will feel when you don't have to face that infernal question—What's for dinner?—six days out of seven.

Option 2: Daily rituals. If you don't like the weekly approach, how about a daily food-prep ritual? Take about twenty or thirty minutes in the morning to get all of your food organized for the day—or do it the night before so you're all set the following day. If you aren't big on cooking, this might consist of simply heading to the salad bar at your local market and loading up a big container with all the food you need.

Option 3: To heck with rituals; have others do it. If your budget allows (and depending on where you live), you could get some of your meals from a service that specializes in healthful, whole-food, plant-based meals. These meals might be delivered or you might have to pick them up, depending on the company.

Whatever approach you take, try to eat as many freshly cooked meals as possible. That may mean taking your lunch to work or school, so here's one last pointer: You don't want your healthful food to make you sick, so be sure to use a cooler or ice packs to keep your food fresh until you're ready to partake. And if you still aren't convinced that it's time to get cookin', just remember, the benefits are directly proportional to the effort you put in. So hey, wait—I do have a mantra for you: "The more you cook, the better you'll look."

Section II:
The Fat Exerciser

Chapter 11
Fat People Exercise Fewer Than Four Hours per Week

> ***If it weren't for the fact that the TV set and the refrigerator are so far apart, some of us wouldn't get any exercise at all.***
>
> —Joey Adams

Let me warn you about a fattitude of the first degree when it comes to exercise: looking at physical activity solely as a way to expend calories. After consuming a rich meal, fat people may punish themselves with hours on the treadmill. They may even avoid forms of exercise they enjoy because those activities "don't burn enough calories." My advice? Turn the dynamic around. When you truly enjoy something, you're more likely to do it. Where exercise is concerned, that means you're more likely to stick with it in the long run, rather than kicking back on the couch watching *America's Next Top Model.*

Why should you even care? Because any attempt to get healthy and fit—and stay that way—will be futile if exercise isn't part of the equation.

Give It Your All—or Even Just 2.5 Percent

One of the most common excuses people offer for not exercising is that they're just "too busy." That's lame. Remember back in the introduction where I discussed the integrity gap and what your schedule says about you? If having a fit body is important to you, exercise is a must. So how much of your precious time do you have to devote to doing a fun physical activity that will enhance your health, well-being, and chances of longevity? A minimum of four hours each week seems to keep people lean.[1–4] If that seems like a lot, it's time to do some math. That boils down to just 2.5 percent of your time (or 3.75 percent, if you're going to be a stickler about how sleep time doesn't count). If having a fit and healthy body isn't worth that much of your time, I'm not sure why you're reading this book.

If there really were one simple (weird, old, or whatever) rule for a flat belly, it would be this: Exercise isn't optional; you need to make time for it day in, day out. Don't leave exercise (or healthful eating) up for debate each day. Trust me, if it's a daily decision, you probably won't do it very often. You've got to make a commitment to yourself and your program and then stick to it. Think about brushing your teeth and flossing. Do you debate the merits of dental hygiene and whether to devote your time to it on a daily basis? I hope not.

Making a commitment is a good starting point, but you've still got to follow through. This is where having fun comes in. Don't turn exercise into drudgery. For that matter, don't tie it to external rewards, like weight loss, recognition from friends, or even fitting into your skinny jeans. External rewards generally aren't sufficient to sustain long-term effort. The reward is in the practice, in living according to your values, and in waking up and feeling great each day. So find a form of exercise you love to do, and then do it because you love it!

Squeezing It In

What's that you say—no time to work out? Break your daily exercise down into several short sessions tied to everyday activities to make sure you get them done. Here's an example of how it might look:

- **Rise and shine—or walk.** Surely you can squeeze in a five-minute walk in the morning—maybe after a cup of green tea but before breakfast? As a bonus, you get to connect with the outdoors, jump-start your metabolism, and maybe even watch the sunrise.
- **Earn your lunch.** Work out the kinks—and work up an appetite—by taking a short walk before lunch.
- **Park it.** When driving to work or running errands, choose a parking space at the far corner of the parking lot, not in front of the door.
- **Cut out early.** If you use public transportation, first and foremost, good for you! Second, get off the bus or subway a few stops early and walk the rest of the way to your destination.
- **Multitask during TV time.** Betcha didn't see this one coming. While I'm not in favor of spending a lot of time in front of the TV or any video screen, chances are you're going to watch anyway. Why not do some crunches or squats or put that cobwebbed, dusty treadmill or exercise bike to use while you watch. This is also a good time to stretch, which always feels good.

Linking activities in this way is one of the best tips I've heard in the past several years. I learned about it in the book *Switch: How to Change When Change Is Hard*, by Chip and Dan Heath. The great thing about this strategy is that it sets your course in advance so you don't have a chance to waffle when the time comes to work out.

Let me tell you about my early years of exercise, back in the mid-1990s. Al Gore was inventing the Internet, *Forrest Gump* was at the top of the box office, my favorite CD was by Alanis Morissette, er, LL Cool J, and I had a workout partner who was also my best friend. Our gym sessions were about working hard and getting in shape for bodybuilding competitions, but just as importantly, we were there to have fun and unwind. We laughed, we lifted, we broke a sweat, we encouraged each other, and, most of all, we looked forward to it. We didn't get crazy about tracking heart rates, monitoring overtraining symptoms, or other technical mumbo jumbo.

That's how I became hooked on exercise (and in case you wonder, yes, I am an exercise junkie). I didn't get the habit because my program was monotonous, overly complicated, and boring, or because it made me fat and prone to rage-fueled crime, like fast food seems to do. Whenever I start feeling stuck in a rut with my workouts, I shake things up and find something new and stimulating to do. I also remind myself why I'm doing it in the first place: because I can, because it's fun, because it feels good, and because it's good for me at every level—including how I conduct myself in the wider world. Alright, I'll admit it outright: I think it makes me a better person.

Just Say No to, Um, Saying No

When people want to chat with me about nutrition and exercise, they're usually feeling fairly motivated to make lifestyle changes. After all, they took the initiative to seek me out, and they're willing to pay for my professional advice. So far, so good. Unfortunately, as we start to explore different ways to achieve their weight-loss and fitness objectives, my suggestions are often promptly rejected, much to my eternal astonishment.

Here's an example: I once had a client whose body fat had accumulated to a whopping 50 percent. Of course she wasn't happy with the situation, so we were trying to formulate a plan for a beginning exercise program. I suggested that she start doing some type of resistance training. I designed a simple ten-minute routine for her to do at home using light weights. Anticipating that she might prefer resisting training to resistance training, I also explained how effective this simple approach could be for her long-term success with weight management, strength and balance

Be honest — does this magnifying glass make my butt look big?
BIZARRO.COM
Dist. by King Features
BIZARROCOMICS.COM
Bizarro, reprinted by permission of Dan Piraro.

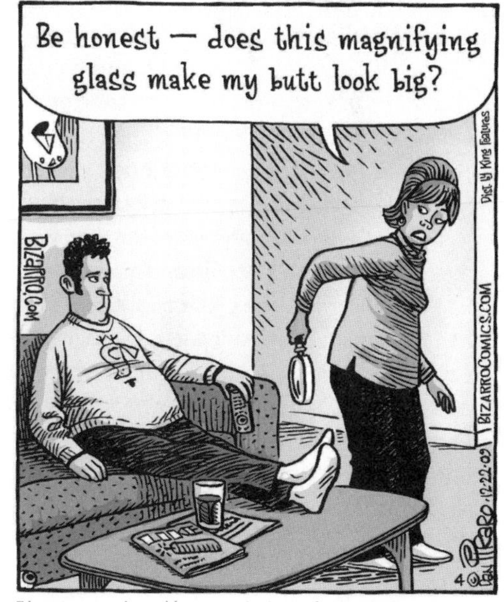

(which help with daily activities and injury prevention), immune function, and so forth. After my big finale, I asked her what she thought. Her response? "I don't like to lift heavy things."

I was speechless. Not for the first time in my professional career, I took a deep breath and silently counted to ten. When she left that day, with the pared-down goal of using a stationary bike two times each week, I was pretty sure that she'd be back in my office a couple of months later, complaining that she wasn't seeing any results from her program.

Resistance Is Not Futile

Please don't be afraid of resistance training. It can be one of the most beneficial things you do for your health and body composition. It doesn't matter if you lift a dumbbell, your own body weight, a jug of water, a stack of books, a small child, or a bag of potting soil. Just do it regularly and with good form. By good form, I mean natural and comfortable movement patterns.

Have you ever seen toddlers squat? They display remarkable form without mirrors or squat machines. They use their leg muscles, stay open at their hips, flare out their toes, and keep their lower backs in a neutral position. Now, have you ever seen out-of-shape fifty-year-olds squat? Yikes! They knock their knees together and round their lower backs so much that they're one bend away from using a spinal disk to play a game of checkers.

Physical movement and exercise should improve your body, not injure it. Too often, people force themselves into strange exercise positions because an infomercial "expert" told them to do it that way. If specific exercises hurt, don't do them. Everyone's body is designed a bit differently. Your legs might be longer than a friend's. Your arms might be shorter than a neighbor's. These mechanical differences matter when you're lifting and moving. If weight lifting makes your shoulders ache, try other upper body exercises that feel more comfortable. If jogging makes your knees hurt, try something else that feels more natural.

If you're a woman and you fear that weight lifting or other forms of resistance training will bulk you up and make you look like Ms. Olympia, well, how can I put this politely . . . the chances are slim to nil that you'll have the discipline to get to that point. (This isn't a gender thing. The vast majority of men don't have the discipline to look like Mr. Olympia either—but the prospect of huge muscles doesn't strike fear in most men's hearts.) But in all seriousness, resistance training can help you shed fat and develop a leaner, toned body without building bulky muscles. For good advice on this topic, check out the excellent articles by Krista Scott-Dixon at her website: stumptuous.com.

Cardio versus Resistance Training

If you're wondering about cardio versus resistance training, I hate to break it to you, but you're living in the past. Let me clear up any confusion on this issue and introduce you to the brave new world of exercise. Classic cardio or aerobic exercises, such as jogging, cycling, and swimming, utilize a lot of energy (calories) and strengthen the heart and lungs. Classic resistance training exercises, such as push-ups, pull-ups, squats, and weight lifting, also utilize a lot of energy (calories) and strengthen the heart and lungs. If you doubt this, do twenty push-ups to experience it firsthand. However, resistance training also has the added benefit of overloading your muscles, and in the long run, that helps preserve them. (If you're still living in the past, I'll let you in on a secret: the reason weight-bearing exercise is so highly touted is because it serves to overload the muscles.)

Conversely, doing only "cardio" exercises doesn't provide enough of an overload to keep muscle on the body. Plus, with repeated, lengthy, intensive bouts of cardio, muscle can become just another fuel source that's gobbled up to sustain the effort. This is a pretty big deal where weight loss is concerned, since muscle is a major regulator of metabolism. And the truth is, it's an important point for everyone, since adequate muscle keeps us functional and active. A natural by-product of aging is muscle loss; we tend to lose about 40 percent of our muscle by age sixty if we don't do resistance training.[5]

Still, when you think of resistance training, you may picture dull, repetitive old-school exercises with long, boring, rest periods between sets. Modern resistance exercise is about keeping things moving with a consistent flow. I recommend that you check out your local gym or maybe even work with a trainer to get up to speed and develop a program that's effective for you.

Just a few words of advice: Before you make a grand plan to focus on resistance training for the next twenty years, remember that doing only one form of exercise, no matter what it is, year after year can lead to injury or burnout. And as your body adapts to that form of exercise, you'll also see diminishing results.

For those who don't like the idea of cardio exercise, I have good news: You can get plenty of lower-intensity cardio exercise simply by using your own body as a means to get around. If you walk to work or around the block after dinner, cycle to the grocery store, and run to catch the bus, spending additional time jogging or cycling is just plain redundant.

Work Harder, Not Smarter

Okay, I admit that it's a little too flip to say, "Work harder, not smarter." Of course I want you to work smart: to devise an exercise regimen that's safe, fun, and effective and that meets your goals. But I also encourage you to keep pushing your limits. Plenty of data indicates that exercising four to five hours each week is imperative for fitness and weight loss. But total exercise time isn't the only thing that matters. The intensity you bring to each workout is also extremely important.[6–9]

Low-intensity aerobic activity is an acceptable form of exercise, and also a good place to start if you're out of shape or haven't been exercising. And no matter where you're at, it's definitely better than nothing. But as you get fitter, add more intensity to your workouts. Need motivation? Just remember that people who work harder tend to be leaner and healthier. I'm not saying you have to fixate on achieving your target heart rate, doing a certain number of reps, or anything like that; I'm just encouraging you to keep pushing your limits. And while I'm not too worried that you're going to go all extreme on me, do keep in mind that it's important to mix in lower-intensity movements, such as yoga, stretching, and walking, to give your connective tissue and nervous system some time to recover.

Be Prepared

Just because you didn't earn a merit badge in sports when you were a scout doesn't mean you can't start now. Always have a backup plan—or three—to ensure that you get some physical activity even when planned workouts don't . . . um . . . work out. Here are some examples:

- Invest in a few fun exercise DVDs. That way if you can't get to the gym, you can always do some yoga, aerobics, or targeted resistance-training exercises.
- Keep a fitness ball at home, at the office, or both. If nothing else, you can sit on it while doing computer work and strengthen your core.
- Set up a pop-up reminder on your computer prompting you to do a few minutes of exercise at strategic moments throughout the day. These bursts of exercise can increase your energy level, so you might even try scheduling them in place of coffee breaks.
- Keep some workout clothes in your backpack, car, or office—or all three. Not having the proper attire is assuredly one of the most lame excuses for not exercising. And if it comes down to it, exercise in whatever you're wearing, as long as you aren't en route to a job interview or dinner with the in-laws.

Mix It Up

Is a sprinter more fit than a bodybuilder? Is a hockey player more fit than an advanced yogi? Is a gymnast more fit than a swimmer? It's hard to say, especially when you consider the various components of fitness, such as cardiovascular endurance, stamina, strength, flexibility, power, coordination, agility, and balance. For optimum fitness, you need to work on all of these areas, which means cross-training. The good news is, this also helps with keeping your program fresh and fun.

To that end, one of my absolute favorite sources for exercise ideas is Monkey Bar Gymnasium (monkeybargym.com), dedicated to full-body training for strength, speed, and stamina. Check it out. But be careful. Side effects include more energy, less body fat, more strength, serious flexibility, and big biceps (if that's what you're looking for). One last thing: Those questions just above, about who's fitter? Let's be real. High-level athletes in any of those sports have a fitness level that vastly exceeds that of the average American. And they all got to be that way by following one simple rule: Just say yes to exercise.

Chapter 12
Fat People Are Lazy

What the country needs are a few labor-making inventions.

—Arnold Glasow

Up to this point, I've talked a lot about eating habits and a bit about exercise. But the fact is, the biggest single factor in being overweight is fattitude, and nowhere is this more obvious than in seemingly innocuous behaviors like riding escalators and elevators, replacing the batteries in the Roomba, lifting a pen to sign a check for the yard guy, or driving to the corner store (probably for a jumbo soft drink and a corndog or two . . . or three . . . or four).

Chop Wood, Carry Water

Have you heard of the Amish? They don't believe in using most forms of newfangled technology. Therefore, they don't spend many hours on the elliptical trainer. Yet they tend to be amazingly fit. Why? Because they do a lot of actual work. They do physical labor in the field and in their homes, and their mode of transportation is often walking. One study showed that, on average, each week Amish men do about ten hours of vigorous work, forty-three hours of moderate physical activity, and twelve hours of walking. This is six times as much physical activity as typical adults from the twelve most modernized nations get. Amish women are also seriously active, recording over fourteen thousand steps a day on a pedometer, compared to just over five thousand for the average American woman. As a result, only 4 percent of the Amish are obese (compared to 31 percent of people in the United States overall) and only 26 percent are overweight (compared to 65 percent of people in the United States overall).[1]

So what does this mean for you? Maybe you need to put down the battery-powered spaghetti-twirling fork, turn off the motorized chocolate milk mixer, and take a page from the Amish. Why not grab a broad-rimmed straw hat and hit the fields—or your front lawn? Instead of buying that automatic ball thrower for your dog, look for opportunities to get physically active, like walking, riding a bike, or taking the stairs. You could even consider doing volunteer work that involves physical labor. That might mean gardening (in your own backyard, in a community garden, or at a local organic farm), picking up litter, coaching for a youth league, or swinging a hammer for Habitat for Humanity. Heck, after getting used to throwing balls for your own dog, you could even throw balls for dogs at the local animal shelter. You'll get more activity and the community will get a new volunteer. It's a win-win situation.

Go Jump in a Lake

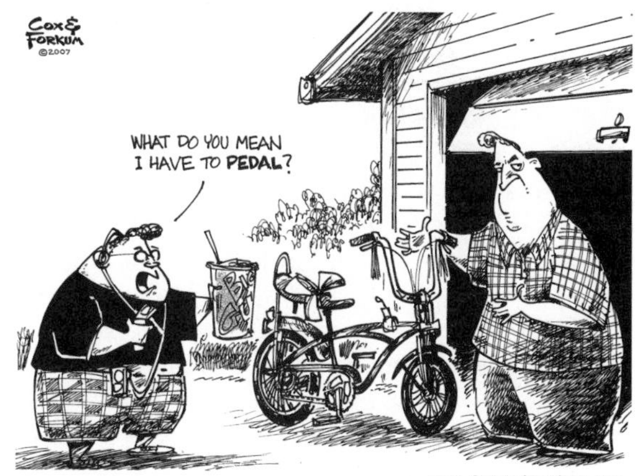

Cox & Forkum ©2007
WHAT DO YOU MEAN I HAVE TO PEDAL?
www.CoxAndForkum.com
Reprinted by permission of Cox and Forkum.

Getting some physical activity each day isn't hard. For example, say you have a desk job. You could schedule three ten-minute walking breaks each day. Better yet, if you work in a multistory building, you could make those stair-climbing breaks. By the end of a five-day workweek, that comes to two and a half hours of exercise. While that definitely isn't Olympic-caliber training, it will tone your body, pump up your metabolism, and maybe even earn you a reputation as a fitness badass at the office.

Beyond hitting the gym or going jogging, what else can you do to up your level of physical activity? Wash windows and push the vacuum cleaner around; it won't kill you (in fact, it will do quite the opposite). Turn up the stereo and dance, play tag with your kids, or pull some weeds—out in the esplanade if your own yard happens to be immaculate. Walk to the store and carry your groceries home, or if you do drive, park as far away from the door as you can. And while I don't advocate watching a TV, I know you're probably going to do it anyway, so why not replace your recliner with a stationary bike? Honestly (and I'm not being rude here), go fly a kite. I mean it: Go for a hike!

All joking aside, the key is to look around you and notice what most North Americans routinely do in terms of physical activity. Then walk in the other direction—vigorously.

Americans generally look at physical labor as a negative thing. We need to flip this around. In today's world, where so many of us spend the vast majority of our waking hours sitting at desks, in cars, or in front of a computer or television, finding more opportunities for physical activity is a bonus. It should be a goal. Seize every opportunity you have to use and challenge your body. Have fun with it and appreciate the fact that an increased activity level will keep your body more fit and functional in the long term.

Make Being Active Make Sense

Being physically active is so rewarding that it should make sense to move your body whenever you get a chance. But your brain may offer some resistance (not the kind of resistance we're looking for here!). Until you build a habit and lifestyle of being more physically active, use whatever means you can to trick your brain into thinking it's a good idea. Here are the kinds of strategies I'm talking about:

- **Gasoline is expensive.** It shouldn't be hard to convince yourself that it makes sense to ride a bike or walk whenever you can—even if that walk is just to the bus stop. Enhance your chances of success by keeping your bike handy on the front porch, learning safe walking routes, and figuring out where the nearest bus stops are.

- **Did I mention that gasoline is expensive?** Ditch the gas-powered mower and use a push mower instead. Added benefits include cleaner air and a tighter butt. Now that's what I call a real win-win. Oh, and by the way, you've heard of those old-fangled inventions called a "rake" and a "broom," right? If you use them instead of a leaf blower, you'll be more buff—*and* earn your neighbors' undying gratitude.

- **De-stress.** The "stress epidemic" may be almost as widespread as the obesity epidemic, and it seems that depression might run a close third. You know what's cool? Physical activity is helpful on all three counts, so when you move your body, you're employing an excellent stress-reduction technique and helping improve your mood and outlook on life.

- **Multitask.** Don't feel like you have enough hours in the day? As the previous point made clear, physical activity is, by its very nature, multitasking. If stress reduction and mood benefits aren't sufficient "accomplishments," you can link physical activity to other goals—maybe as concrete as using that push mower, and maybe broader, like spending quality time with your kids while playing outdoors.

- **Walk your talk.** This might just be the ultimate multitasking win-win. Why not have walking meetings with colleagues? Note that you'll earn an extra gold star if you employ this strategy because you'll also be helping others develop a more active lifestyle.

The ability to be active is one of those things people tend to take for granted—until they get injured, too old, or, yes, too fat too move their bodies. Unfortunately, at that point it may be very difficult to turn the situation around, or maybe even too late.

It may be trite, but I'm going to say it anyway: Use it or lose it. Imagine waking up every day and enjoying the opportunity to be active and move around. Then turn that dream into reality.

Section III: The Fat Life

Chapter 13
Fat People Don't Get Enough Sleep

A good laugh and a long sleep are the best cures in the doctor's book.

—Irish proverb

Here's a shocking statistic: As many as one in four people are too tired to have sex.[1] Folks, if you're too tired for a roll in the hay, my crystal ball says you won't be hitting the gym for a workout anytime soon. But you know what's really sad about this story? Most of us get too little sleep by choice, not necessity. Late nights in front of the TV, computer, or game console (or the fridge) tend to cut into your shut-eye and, as a result, perhaps your energy for the horizontal hustle—you know, the mattress mambo? Worse, being fatigued can feed into a vicious cycle of fatness in a number of ways,[2,3] including impairing your ability to make less-than-crappy food choices.

A century ago, the average American got nearly nine hours of sleep each night. Now the average adult is getting about seven hours of sleep per night, and one-third of Americans sleep less than six and a half hours per night. In addition, nearly six in ten people report that when they do sleep, they don't sleep well.[1] Among my clients who are overweight and have lifestyle-related health problems, I would estimate that nine out of ten don't get sufficient sleep.

Drop and Give Me Forty (Winks, That Is)

Experts agree that sleep is crucial to good health. In the long term it can be as important for overall health as diet and exercise. If you doubt this, consider that people can only survive about eleven days when totally deprived of sleep.[4] Most Americans are living proof that you can survive a lot longer than that without exercise—and most Americans could probably live off of their fat stores alone for at least eleven *weeks*.

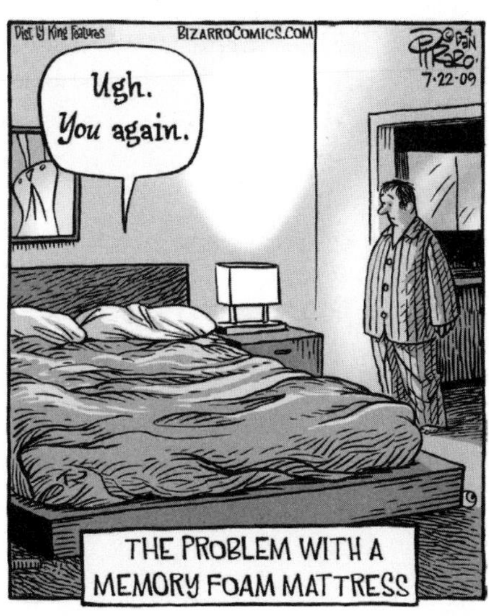

Bizarro, reprinted by permission of Dan Piraro.

Still think that missing out on a few Zs is no big deal? Studies have determined that going twenty-four hours without sleep impairs your functioning on par with a blood alcohol level of 0.10 percent. That's way over the legal limit for driving in most countries, and for good reason. At that point, reflexes, reaction time, and motor control are out the window, and most people are prone to staggering and slurred speech. Going without sleep for twenty-one hours produces changes akin to a 0.08 percent blood alcohol concentration—still over the legal limit in most countries. Even just staying awake for as few as three extra hours can impair the ability to maintain speed and road position while driving.[5, 6]

"Interesting," you say. "But how does this relate to being fat and unhealthy?" Well, if you're a danger to yourself on the road, do you really think you're going to do much better at navigating the aisles at the grocery store, the menu of the local fast-food joint, or even the shelves of your refrigerator? Call it a hunch, but I'm guessing your food selections won't be stellar.

Still, some people proudly proclaim how well they function with only minimal time in the land of Nod. I think they're fooling themselves—and ignoring the stakes. Beyond resulting in poor food choices, too little sleep can lead to lack of energy, wacky blood sugar levels, weight gain, type 2 diabetes, and a chaotic appetite.[3, 7–12] Not good for your waistline—or your life line. If looking good, feeling good, and living longer don't provide sufficient motivation for you to get enough sleep, you might also consider the bottom line: think about how your medical bills could increase.

Hungry Hormones

The list of health issues related to insufficient sleep is alarming—and fairly extensive. How can sleep have such far-reaching influences? It has to do with hormones. When you don't get enough sleep, levels of growth hormone decrease and levels of cortisol increase. The name "growth hormone" may make you think that this metabolic messenger will just make you get bigger and bigger, but that isn't what it does. It helps tissues rebuild and frees up stored fat for use as an energy source.

Cortisol, which is elevated during times of stress, tends to have the opposite effect. It means well; it's trying to ensure that you have energy to fight off an attacker, or at least run like hell, and one way it does so is by breaking down protein to free up amino acids for conversion to glucose. While this is great in situations that are actually dangerous, chronically elevated cortisol damages the body in a number of ways. Where does the protein come from that cortisol causes to be converted to glucose? Your muscles! Combine low levels of growth hormone with elevated cortisol, and you may just end up looking like Jabba the Hutt.

And then there's ghrelin, a hormone that's a dieter's worst nightmare—waking nightmare, that is. Ghrelin stimulates the appetite and makes you want to eat. And the shorter your sleep duration, the higher your ghrelin levels. This is an important point, so let me spell it out for you: Less sleep means more ghrelin, and more ghrelin means more appetite.[9, 12] Unfortunately, you won't be likely to gorge on foods like kale and strawberries. Less sleep usually leads to cravings for calorie-dense, nutrient-poor foods. Hello cupcakes, candy bars, and fried pies!

Now let me introduce you to my good buddy leptin. If ghrelin is like the Wicked Witch of the East, you can think of the hormone leptin as your fairy godmother. One of its functions is to control appetite, and—wonder of wonders—levels of leptin tend to decline when you don't get enough sleep.

Your Ticket to Slumberland

Are you starting to see a trend yet? As a coach, I am, and in real life, not just studies. Sleepy people look at me with sleepy, confused faces and don't understand why they have forty-inch waists.

If you aren't getting seven to nine hours of sleep each night, make it a high priority to turn this situation around. As with any area of life that relates to your long-term health, this is not a place to offer excuses. Yes, we live in a busy world. No, you need not be a victim of it. You still get to choose how you spend your time.

If you take medication, talk with your doctor to determine whether it could be interfering with your sleep and, if so, whether there are other options. You may also need to work with your doctor to rule out other physical causes of sleep problems. Still, there are plenty of things that anyone can do to increase the chances of a good night's sleep. Here are just a few:

- Avoid caffeine, stimulants, and nicotine. If you do consume caffeine, make sure you do so before noon.
- Drink alcohol in moderation, if at all, and never just before bedtime.
- Try to stick to a regular schedule for going to bed and getting up.
- Don't take naps.
- Exercise at least four hours per week (but not late in the evening).
- Keep your bedroom quiet, dark, and comfortable.
- Eat real food and avoid getting overly full before bed.
- Don't watch TV or use the computer just before bed.
- Get outdoors every day.
- Meditate or practice relaxation techniques before bed.

All of these guidelines are easy enough to follow, so motivation shouldn't be an issue. But if it is, consider this: people who get enough sleep also tend to have healthy relationships, adequate social support, and a career they are content with. Sleep helps you feel more positive, and that tends to breed more positivity.

Chapter 14
Fat People Use Food to Manage Their Feelings

I can't stop eating. I eat because I'm unhappy, and I'm unhappy because I eat. It's a vicious cycle.

—Fat Bastard, in Austin Powers: The Spy Who Shagged Me

Did you know that people who suffer from depression have very low levels of stimulation? They don't tend to get a lot of fresh air, sunlight, exercise, human contact, and so forth. Not surprisingly, when people are understimulated, they seek . . . umm . . . stimulation. What can provide quick and easy stimulation without leaving the house, and with no questions asked? Food. Food can temporarily ease depression and elevate levels of various "feel good" neurotransmitters in the brain.[1,2] This makes me think that one of the reasons people tend to overeat, and especially tend to eat so much processed food, is because their lives are boring and unstimulating. To be honest, this issue might trump all the others.

More Awesomeness, Please

Here's an inverse relationship that holds true for many people:

- When life stimulation goes up, consumption of junk food goes down.
- When life stimulation goes down, consumption of junk food goes up.

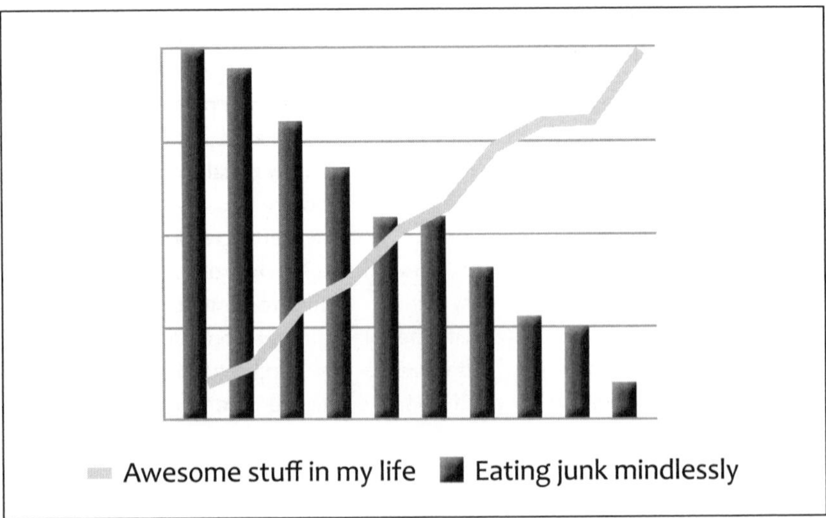

Thanks to Krista Scott-Dixon (stumptuous.com) for this image.

Have you noticed this? If you have a thriving and challenging career, engaging relationships, exciting hobbies, plenty of physical activity, adequate time outdoors, satisfying volunteer activities, and so on, life feels full and stimulating. When your job is boring, your family is bumming you out, and you don't have anything to get excited about, you may seek to fill the void with junk food. Unfortunately, that can be a gargantuan void, and the correspondingly massive intake of junk food can leave you looking like the Pillsbury Doughboy.

If you turn to food for stimulation once in a while, it probably isn't a big deal. But when it becomes a way of life, it's definitely a problem. And let's get real: crappy food is typically the source of the problem. If you're eating for stimulation or to change you're mood, I bet you're reaching for the chocolate or ice cream, not broccoli or lentils.

But what I find really fascinating is what happens next: When people realize that they're eating a lot of crappy food, feeling horrible, and getting ever fatter, what do they do? They usually begin to focus on food (or exercise), even more. They diet, they count calories, they weigh their food, they read weight-loss tips, and so on. But in reality, the problem isn't food; the problem is life. These folks lack engaging daily activities, satisfying relationships, and all the things that feed us in other ways. It's kind of like feeling down and taking an antidepressant instead of taking a good look at your situation and the root of the problem. You can mask your feelings with food, but they won't change until you make changes in your life.

Reality ~~Bites~~ Gorges

In my professional life, I work with a lot of people who eat compulsively. The first question I ask these folks is "Are you getting enjoyment and pleasure from other areas of life?" Because until that happens, these people are probably going to continue to seek solace in food.

People who have undergone gastric bypass surgery tend to be an extreme (and very sad) example of this. They're usually compliant with their new dietary restrictions for a few months, but by the time their one-year post-op rolls around, they've often started gaining weight again. Why? Because food was never the problem; life was. If they don't address life issues, they usually end up turning to food again, no matter how small their stomach is.

I remember chatting with an overweight client after working with her for three months. She wasn't making progress, and she felt discouraged. I asked her to think about why she kept eating so much junk food when doing so didn't match up with her supposed values. She came back with a very insightful response: She told me she was eating junk food at work each day because she hated her job. Her work was boring and tedious, and candy, snacks, and soda helped her get through the day.

So ask yourself: If you struggle with overeating, have you figured out the real reason why you eat when you aren't hungry? Does your junk food consumption go down in proportion to how stimulating and satisfying your life is?

News Flash: It Isn't All about You

Hopefully you've made some changes based on what you've read up to this point in the book. Hopefully you're exercising and sleeping more and making more conscious choices about what, when, where, how, and even why you're eating. After all, it all comes down to you. Or does it? I don't want to be flip here, because everything you've read thus far in this book is extremely important for weight loss. But now I'm going to give you one of my top tips for getting fit, and you're probably going to think I'm nuts. Regardless, here goes: The best way to get fit is to feel happy, and the best way to feel happy is to make someone else happy.

I'm serious. When people focus on their own lives, and particularly on their problems, they tend to get self-centered and negative. I recommend inverting that equation. When you go out of your way to put others first, you'll be rewarded with satisfaction, contentment, and happiness. As author and holistic health counselor Victoria Moran says, "Ease someone else's burden, and yours gets a little lighter."[3] Give it a try and see for yourself.

Don't fall for the fattitude that getting lean is the key to happiness. It simply isn't true that once you're thinner, you'll surely be a happier or better person. The number on the scale is fairly arbitrary, and it doesn't say much about what's in your heart or your mind.

Still, this line of thought is a double-edged sword, since many people could substantially improve their quality of life by losing weight. I think it comes down to perspective. You can spend years playing the game of dieting, focusing on food, and trying to lose weight as a distraction from problems in other areas of your life. Alternatively, you can focus on your values and who you want to be and then use your successes in weight loss and fitness as a stepping-stone to implementing other changes in your life. Allen Zadoff put it well in his book *Hungry: Lessons Learned on the Journey from Fat to Thin*: "I looked at my history and saw clearly that diets and exercise did not work for me. I was trying to change my outsides; while my problem was inside . . . I focused on my emotional and spiritual development. I put 10 percent of my energy into eating and 90 percent into spiritual and emotional healing. When I changed my focus, I found my body was restored to normal proportions over time. I didn't lose weight because I tried to lose weight. Weight loss occurred as a by-product of working on other things."[4]

The bottom line? Weight loss and body transformation is a somewhat superficial goal (and one the diet industry counts on). If we would all devote some of that energy, focus, and commitment to helping others and making the world a better place, imagine how powerful that would be.

Food Addiction and Escapism

You've undoubtedly noticed that I've alluded to an addiction to fast food or processed food a few times in this book. You may be a little skeptical about this claim. So let's back up and take a look at the definition of addiction, in this case from *Merriam-Webster's 11th Collegiate Dictionary*: "Compulsive need for and use of a habit-forming substance (as heroin, nicotine, or alcohol) characterized by tolerance and by well-defined physiological symptoms upon withdrawal; broadly: persistent compulsive use of a substance known by the user to be harmful."

According to that definition, I am 99.999 percent positive that food addiction exists. How many people do you know who consistently eat too much health-degrading food even though they know it's harmful to their health and well-being? I rarely meet people who don't do this.

As a society, we tend to accept and even encourage food addiction. You've assuredly heard food advertisements with slogans like "can't get enough," "nobody can say no," or "can't eat just one." What if we had those kinds of advertisements for other addictive substances, like alcohol? Oh wait—we do have advertisements for alcohol. Hmm, maybe that explains why the third leading lifestyle-related cause of death in the United States is excessive alcohol consumption.[5]

Although that sort of proves my point, let's consider what would happen if we had advertisements encouraging and glamorizing the use of heroin or crack cocaine, and even insinuating just how much better your life would be if you'd just drop a few bucks at your local den of iniquity on a daily basis. People would be outraged. They'd be protesting 24/7. But somehow promoting foods that decimate our health is not only permitted, it's actually the foundation of a huge sector of our economy.

When you think of addictive foods, which ones come to mind? I'd bet dollar to doughnuts (oops! was doughnuts one of them?) that you thought of cakes, cookies, chips, fast food, or cheese. I have yet to meet anyone who claims to be "addicted" to pinto beans, kale, or pears. Food addiction is a problem that wouldn't exist (or would only exist in rare cases) if it weren't for major food companies creating foods that are "irresistible" to the consumer. Foods that occur in nature usually don't possess addictive qualities.

This probably won't come as huge news to you, but avoiding pain through any addiction, whether to drugs, alcohol, nicotine, or food, isn't a workable solution. Sometimes life is painful, and we need to accept that and learn to experience the pain and cope with it in positive ways. In the end, what destroys us isn't the pain we encounter in life; it's how we relate to that pain and what we do with it. And there's no surer path to self-defeat than addiction.

If any of this strikes a chord for you, you may be wondering how you can learn to deal with life's pain. My recommendation is that you practice putting yourself in slightly painful situations. When you stretch yourself and get out of your comfort zone, that small dose of pain will help you build tolerance.

I'm not saying you need to hit your thumb with a hammer, sit through a production of Wagner's entire *Der Ring des Nibelungen*, or go to your ex's wedding. Start small: When you tolerate some hunger between meals, that's pain. When you add five minutes to your workout time, that's pain. When you stretch further in yoga class, that's pain. These kinds of experiences can be like a "pain vaccination," building resilience that will help support and protect you when life gets tough. Then, when painful life events do inevitably arise, look at them as an opportunity to flex your coping muscles, rather than a chance to cave in to addictions.

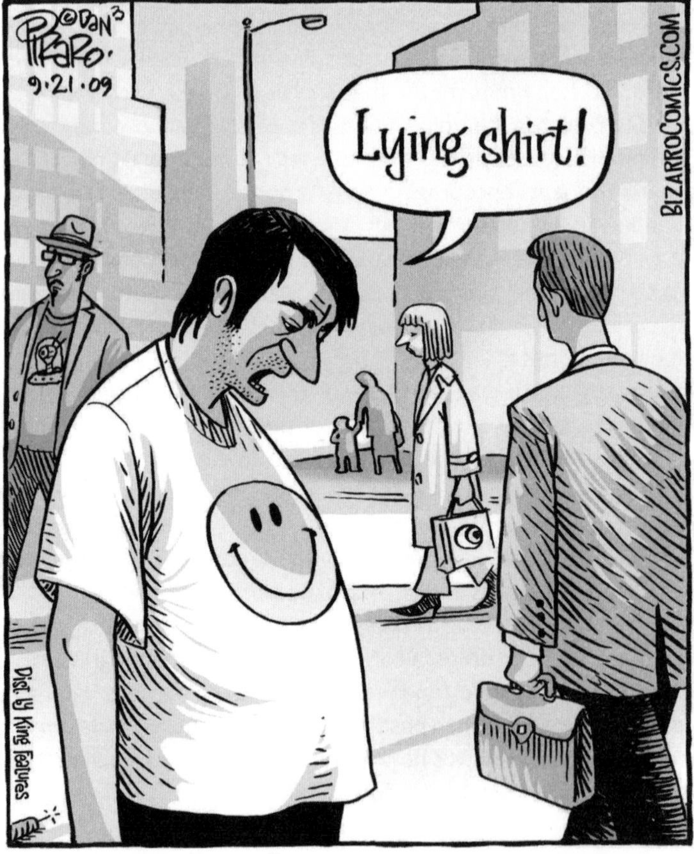

Bizarro, reprinted by permission of Dan Piraro.

Chapter 15
Fat People Put Themselves in Fat-Inducing Situations

Wisdom is the quality that keeps you from getting into situations where you need it.

—Doug Larson

It's time for another pop quiz. Take a look at these situations and try to visualize the people they apply to:

- They have lots of cookies and chips in their pantry.
- They have to drive fifteen minutes to get to the closest gym, park, or recreation center.
- They have a credit card—and know how to use it.
- They have cable TV.
- They have a candy dish on their desk.
- They drive everywhere—even to the next-door neighbor's.
- They hang out with people who drink and stay up late.

Now, be honest: Did you visualize people who are lean, fit, and happy? Or did you maybe visualize people who are overweight, unhealthy, in debt, and unhappy?

Situation Normal

So, what should these theoretical people do? It's tough. Even though the logical brain knows that it's important to save for retirement, the emotional brain often wants to buy, buy, buy, even if it means maxing out the credit card. The emotional brain can be hard to resist. The solution? Don't get a credit card.

Likewise, the logical brain knows that it's best to eat just a cookie or two. Unfortunately, the emotional brain wants to eat four or five. . . . Okay, just one more. . . . Okay, just one more, and this time I really mean it! The solution? Don't keep a bunch of cookies around.

The situations we put ourselves in can be life altering—even for someone like me, with a life based on health and fitness. I know my tendencies, and I know that I can't rely on willpower alone. It might get me through tough circumstances every once in awhile—but daily? No way. When I put myself in tempting or negative situations, it leads to one thing: failure. You may find this hard to believe, so let me be honest with you and tell you what my crystal ball says I would do if I were one of those hypothetical people profiled above—and how I'd set myself up to avoid failure:

- If I had lots of cookies and chips in my pantry, I'd probably eat lots of cookies and chips. Instead, I keep veggies, beans, fruits, whole grains, nuts, and seeds on hand.
- If I had to drive fifteen minutes to the gym, I probably wouldn't go to the gym very often. So I make sure to set up residence in close proximity to a gym.
- If I had a credit card, I'd probably buy stuff I can't really afford and be in debt. Instead, I pay with cash.
- If I had cable TV, I'd probably be mesmerized and stay up late watching sitcoms, B movies, and eventually infomercials. Instead, I stick to reading and occasionally watching DVDs.
- If I had a candy dish on my desk, I'd probably eat candy all day. Instead, I keep a variety of green and herbal teas on hand.
- If I had a car, I'd probably be tempted to drive everywhere, eventually even to the gym! Instead, I walk, bicycle, and use mass transit.
- If I hung out with people who drink and stay up late, I'd probably do the same. Instead, I have friends who value their health and choose to exercise and eat nutritious foods. I like having friends who are fitter than I am or have a more healthful lifestyle; this challenges me to become a better person.

As a dietitian and coach, I frequently meet people who put themselves in situations that don't align with their values (or at least what they claim to value). This may sound harsh, but I'm usually pretty sure that they aren't going to meet their fitness goals. And you know what? That's alright—it's their choice. But they do need to accept that this is the probable outcome and not anticipate anything different. They need to understand that setting themselves up for failure is the biggest fattitude of all.

Sure, some people have great self-discipline and can maintain healthful habits even when they put themselves in challenging situations. But this generally isn't sustainable in the long run. What we do is usually based on how we construct our lives. Why tempt fate or make things more difficult? Instead, put yourself in situations that align with your values and goals. This makes positive behaviors more effortless.

Imitation Is the Sincerest Form of Fattery

A wise man once said, "All television is educational television. The question is: what is it teaching?"[1] My opinion? I think it's teaching fattitudes. TV food advertisements aren't pushing healthful food. Nine of every ten food ads during good old Saturday morning cartoons are for absolute crap—or, to be more precise, "foods high in fat, sodium, or added sugars, or low in nutrients."[2] Horrors! Does this mean that toaster pastries and chocolate puffed cereals aren't healthful? But all joking aside, this is a serious issue. Kids are impressionable, and they usually aren't able to distinguish between healthful food and junk food. And even if they can, they may lack the perspective to understand why a healthful diet is important or lack the willpower to resist advertisements designed to appeal to them.

You may think that television is innocuous—perhaps a waste of time, but hardly insidious. But I think watching TV just might be the triple threat of fattitudes—and the ultimate fat-inducing situation. Think about it: TV time typically takes the place of doing things that are more active. People tend to eat while watching. And based on my observations of what grocery carts are typically filled with, I know that most people are influenced by TV food advertising. If all of that doesn't convince you to turn off the TV, here's one last tidbit to chew on: We humans tend to imitate each other, and behaviors can be contagious. What you see people eating on TV can influence what you decide to eat, and this can occur at the conscious or subconscious level.

Leaving Normal

If you've been paying attention as you read this book, or even if you've just been paying attention in the parking lot at your local warehouse store, you are no doubt aware that for most Americans, fattitude is everything—and then some. Therefore, choosing a healthful lifestyle and placing yourself in situations that support your goals may mean setting a new social norm.

The Joy of Tech™
by Nitrozac & Snaggy
HAH HAH! LOOK AT THE NEW KID, HIS BODY MASS INDEX IS EASILY UNDER THE 95TH PERCENTILE!
HE PROBABLY DOES SPORTS AND STUFF, INSTEAD OF WATCHING TV AND PLAYING VIDEO GAMES! DUMBASS!
I BET WHEN HE LOOKS DOWN, HE CAN SEE HIS FEET! WEIRDO!
YOU COULD FIT TWO OF HIM IN MY JEANS! IDIOT!
©2008 Geek Culture
joyoftech.com
Thanks to geekculture.com for this cartoon.

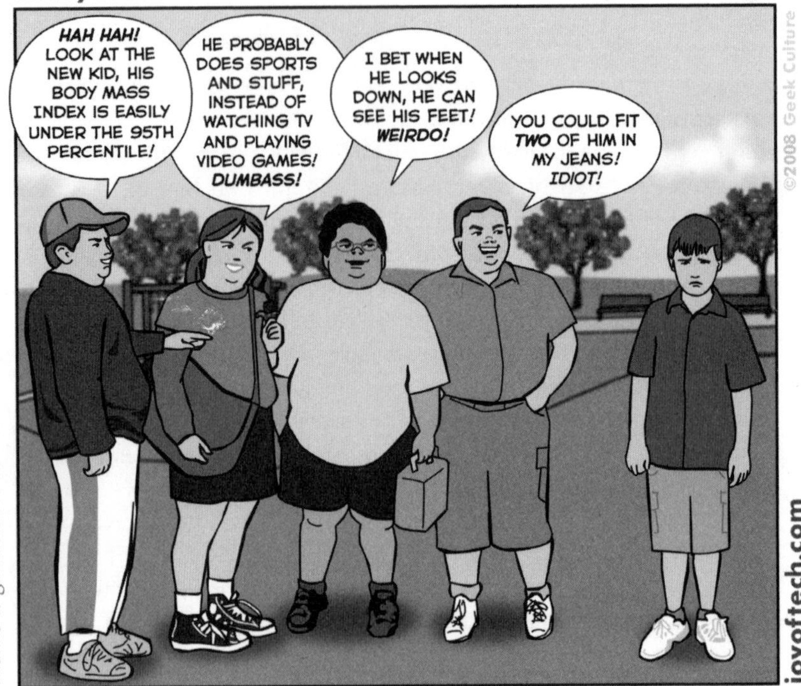

Fat kids, the new norm.

Don't Be a Rotten Apple on the Family Tree

Let me tell you a heartwarming story. Once upon a time I was babysitting my nephews, who were four and two years old at the time. When mealtime rolled around, they provided me with a valuable insight about how eating habits develop: When young kids see someone eat, they immediately want the same food.

Here's what happened: I asked the four-year-old if he wanted any vegetables. His reply was a forceful "No!" Three minutes later I brought some raw veggies and salad dressing to the table and started to eat them. He immediately changed his tune, and it was music to my ears: "Uncle Ryan, I want veggies and salad dressing!" Then, about forty-five seconds later, he exclaimed that veggies and salad dressing were his favorite food combination.

A few minutes later I asked the two-year-old if he wanted anything else to eat and received another emphatic "No!" Three minutes later I brought a banana to the table that I was going to eat. He too changed his tune, reaching out a hand and exclaiming "Nana!" (Translation: "Uncle Ryan, give me your banana and fend for yourself!") As he made short work of the banana, some scary thoughts crossed my mind. What if I had pathetic nutrition habits? What if I'd brought a bag of fast food or a box of cupcakes to the table? That's what the kids would have wanted, mainly because I was eating it. If they saw me eating it, they would think it was "normal" food.

Then I realized that some parents bring crappy food into the house day after day, year after year, which gave me a little more sympathy for thirty-something clients who can't seem to quit eating junk. They are victims of their social norm—and worse, their family norm. Talk about being set up for failure!

To give you an idea of just how much family matters, consider the results of a study of eighteen hundred children who were tracked from before birth until age four. It identified the following factors as major predictors of early childhood obesity:[3]

- Fat moms
- Minimal breast-feeding
- Introducing solid foods before four months of age
- Less sleep time during infancy
- TV in the child's bedroom
- Higher intake of fast food
- Drinking more sugar-sweetened beverages

While it may seem fairly obvious that our parents have an enormous effect on us, distant relatives can also have a surprising impact. Family members thousands of miles away can actually influence a person's body weight. Research indicates that seeing an obese relative just once per year can reset a person's expectations about acceptable body size.[4]

And if you ever doubted how important it is to lead by example, consider that an article in the prestigious *New England Journal of Medicine* concluded that obesity appears to spread through social networks.[5] So when you plan your next family gathering or get-together, you might want to opt for something a little more active than a Monopoly tournament.

The Nut Doesn't Fall Far from the Tree

Here's a sample of a conversation I often have with fairly new clients:

Client: "Ryan, I keep eating junk food, and it's preventing me from reaching my weight-loss and fitness goals."

Me: "Tell me why you're still eating junk food."

Client: "Well, I just kept thinking about that pint of ice cream in the freezer and . . ."

Me: "Wait a minute! You had ice cream at your house? Remember how we discussed the importance of setting yourself up for success by surrounding yourself with nutritious whole foods?"

Client: "But Ryan, I have two kids. They can eat ice cream, and they want to eat it. I *have* to keep it in the house for them."

At this point in the conversation, I often have to take a deep breath and count to ten. But since you aren't sitting in my office, I'll go ahead and tell you what I think: I don't care if you're fat, thin, young, or old. I don't care if you're an exercise fanatic or a couch potato. No one should be consuming junk food on a regular basis—end of discussion. If processed food is all your kids or spouse will eat, drop them off on a deserted island for two months and see what happens. If you haven't had much to eat for a couple days, fresh fruit and wild greens look pretty darn good. People will eat nutritious foods when they're hungry.

If someone in your household loves ice cream (or whatever) and insists on having it, tell them to go out and have an ice cream cone and be done with it. You don't have to stock up on gallon buckets of the stuff. The idea that you need to keep junk food in the house for other family members is a bunch of BS. Don't cop out and play the family card because you're ambivalent about changing your own diet. And remember, good nutrition is important for everyone, not just people who are trying to lose weight.

Change is hard. Changing your very identity is even harder. Don't sabotage your health-related goals just to please others. You may be afraid you'll lose friends or offend family members if you get in shape and leave them in the fat lane. But think of it this way: the life you save may be your own. And if it's true that the best way to lead is by example, then maybe you'll be saving their lives too.

Chapter 16
Fat People Are All-or-None Thinkers

There is no black-and-white situation. It's all part of life: highs, lows, middles.

—Van Morrison

Sometimes when I do lectures, I have the audacity to mention that popcorn is a whole grain, and that potatoes have a low calorie density. As if that weren't shocking enough, I even have the hubris to suggest that popcorn and potatoes are both fine options in a whole-food, plant-based approach to controlling body fat. Audiences tend to gasp aloud, and afterward they're all abuzz about how they're going to start eating popcorn and potatoes all day, "because it's good for them."

This kind of thinking makes me crazy. What gave people the idea that popcorn was unhealthful? Why did they think potatoes would make them fat? Maybe the bigger question is, why are people inclined to see things in such an extreme light, labeling certain foods as "good" or "bad"? Once these tidy little categories are established, the next thing you know people are fastidiously avoiding fat, shrinking in fear from carbohydrates, or trying to get by eating only cabbage soup or grapefruit. Not a day goes by that I don't get questions about whether a certain nutrition bar is healthful, if dried fruit is terrible, if fat-free deli slices are the answer, or if bread is the devil's handiwork. People want a black-and-white answer. They want me to decree whether the food is good or bad, healthful or unhealthful.

Only Shades of Gray

As with everything in life, all foods lie somewhere on a spectrum. Some are better, and some are worse. Some foods have more health benefits, and some have fewer. And in addition to the food itself, you have to consider how much of it you're eating, not to mention how, why, when, where, and with whom you're eating. But in the end, perhaps the most important questions is, what's the alternative? What would you be eating instead? Let's look at a few examples.

"Ryan, is store-bought rotisserie chicken good?"
—What's the alternative?

- Is organic, free-range chicken, prepared at home better? Yes, slightly.
- Would kale and lentils be way better? Definitely.
- Is a fast-food fried chicken sandwich worse? Yes, totally.

Bottom line: The rotisserie chicken is better than some options, but worse than others.

"Ryan, are freeze-dried veggies healthful to snack on?"
—What's the alternative?

- If you're going to eat freeze-dried veggies instead of cheese crackers from a vending machine, we have a winner.
- If you're eating freeze-dried veggies instead of raw or freshly cooked veggies, that's probably a step in the wrong direction.

Bottom line: The freeze-dried veggies are better than some options, but worse than others.

"Ryan, I'm a raw-vegan mom, and when my son goes to his father's house on the weekends cooked squash is served for dinner!"
—What's the alternative?
Bottom line: If the worst part of your kid's diet is cooked squash, you don't have much to worry about in the world of nutrition.

I'll have number 7.
I'll have a wide assortment of ingredients from your menu, in different combinations than you offer them, but first, this series of probing questions.
BIZARROCOMICS.COM
©DAN PIRARO 2-25-10
BIZARRO.COM
Bizarro, reprinted by permission of Dan Piraro.

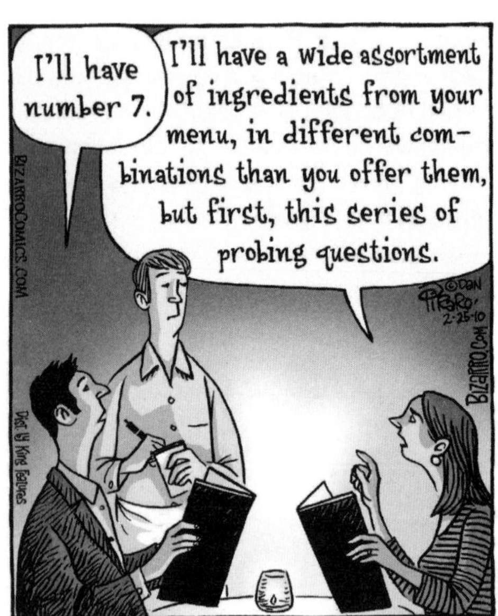

Taboo Foods

What about taboo foods? Many people have a list of foods they consider unhealthful—things they won't let themselves eat, even as they reach for another single-serve fat-free pudding. Let's take a look at some foods that have been demonized and what they can tell us about trying to put food into black-and-white categories:

Bread. If you think of bread as akin to a gateway drug or tend to find yourself going for that fifth slice of raisin toast, I'm guessing that you buy the standard bread that lines the shelves of supermarkets, made with refined flour, sweeteners, preservatives, and possibly a long list of unpronounceable ingredients. The answer? Try buying a loaf of sprouted-grain bread and eating a slice of it plain. It's tasty, but it's not *too* tasty. You won't find yourself mowing through a loaf anytime soon. Sprouted-grain bread is essentially a whole food, and it's very satisfying and nutritious.

Burritos. Sure, burritos can be scary when made with mounds of white rice, lard-infused beans, fatty beef, and a heap of processed cheese. But if you start with a sprouted or whole-grain tortilla and fill it with veggies, beans, salsa, and avocado, you're golden.

Cookies. Cookies are an indulgence; no doubt about that. But the real problem is the white flour, sugar, and butter or margarine they usually contain. When made with whole-grain flour, fruit, nuts, and moderate amounts of unrefined sweeteners and vegetable oil, a cookie can actually be a nutritional powerhouse.

Pizza. True, pizza is a dietary disaster when loaded with fatty cheeses and meats. Plus, a commercial whole-grain crust is about as common as a North American choosing to take the stairs: very rare. But a homemade pizza on a whole-grain crust, with chunky tomato sauce and loads of veggies? Sounds like a winner to me.

Popcorn. Popcorn does have an ugly side—and unfortunately it's the one most folks are familiar with: standard movie theater fare and most microwave varieties, coated in butter, salt, sugar, or cheese. But popcorn is a whole grain, and when it's air popped or popped in a little vegetable oil, it's a great choice.

Potatoes. Folks, a potato is simply a humble root vegetable—until you drown it in butter, cheese, bacon, sour cream, or salt—or all of the above. On its own, a 6-ounce potato clocks in at about 150 calories. Let me pull out my calculator. Hmm, that means you'd need to eat about five pounds of potatoes to rack up 2,000 calories. Good luck with that!

The Biggest Loser

When people struggle with their weight, the all-or-none mentality usually extends beyond individual foods to eating in general. People seem to think that if they aren't 100 percent on a diet, they might as well be 100 percent off a diet. I'm impressed when people transition from eating compulsively to following a perfectly outlined diet plan—but I'm also wary. All too often, obsessing about whether or not to have a side of rice with dinner or a piece of fruit for a snack leads folks down the primrose path to nutritional failure. After a few days of deprivation, they give in to a craving and—voilà!—disgusted at their failure to stick to the plain, they throw their hands up in despair and go on a taquito bender.

This might not be such a big deal for a few days, but what if it turns into monthlong binge session? Bad news: One study showed that a four-week period of excessive fast-food intake coupled with minimal physical activity resulted in increased fat mass as much as two and a half years later.[1] That's right: Using the all-or-none approach to justify bingeing actually could mean higher cholesterol and tight pants a year or two later.

Here's an idea: How about eating three reasonable, healthful meals a day, and a snack if you're genuinely hungry, and not obsessing about the small stuff? In my experience, the people who succeed in weight loss—and in life—are those who have learned to navigate the gray area between "all" and "none." Trying to slavishly stick to a restrictive diet (and beating yourself up when you inevitably fail) isn't the answer. The key is to consistently make smarter choices and build momentum for moving in a positive direction. Don't think of it as being like climbing Mount Everest; think of it as taking a series of small steps. After all, that's how you ultimately get to the top of Mount Everest anyway.

And in case you wondered: Yes, this applies to exercise too. Just because you can't do high-intensity exercise sixty minutes every day of the year doesn't mean you have to settle for zero minutes of exercise most every day. Why not find a few fun physical activities that you can enjoy doing for twenty to thirty minutes, three times per week? And if you happen to miss a few days, or even a few weeks, how about not giving up? Remember, each day offers you the opportunity to get back on track. Just say yes to reasonable, achievable goals.

Chapter 17
Fat People Focus on Short-Term Gain (Literally!)

Consequences are unpitying.
—George Eliot

As discussed in chapter 14, our relationships with food often have a hefty emotional component, and emotions tend to value immediate gains (like a massive dessert or fatty steak) at the cost of future expenses (body fat, heart disease, destruction of our planet's resources, and so forth). The emotional brain adores the prospect of an immediate reward, but it doesn't really comprehend the link with weight gain or disease, and it doesn't necessarily fall in line behind a concept like stopping eating because we're full. When the emotional brain is in charge, food impulses don't encounter much resistance. We eat whatever we want, and however much of it we want, and leave the consequences until later.

Same Old, Same Old

A few years back I read an interesting title in the *Journal of the American Dietetic Association*: "A Descriptive Study of Past Experiences with Weight-Loss Treatment."[1] In this study, researchers examined experiences with weight-loss treatment and treatment preferences among people with ongoing, long-term weight issues. While this study promised to shed some light on how overweight people think, I had to wonder if it could really offer any startling insights. After all, Americans have been fighting (and losing) the battle of the bulge for quite a while now.

In my job as a fitness coach, I sometimes feel like I've heard it all when it comes to people's experiences, preferences, and—yes—excuses. And of course I feel like I have the answers, which is why I've written this book. Still, if you're in the same (capsizing) boat as those interviewed for the study, you might benefit from having a look at how fat people think about weight loss, and why the typical approach doesn't work.

Researchers' question: What is the preferred method of weight-loss for people who are overweight?

Participants' response: Over 93 percent of the people interviewed said they had previously tried to lose weight by "doing it on their own," and this method remained the most popular, being the top choice of over 30 percent of those responding.

My comment: This may stem from a need for control. That's cool. I'm all for using your own experience to make gradual changes and not needing a diet coach to dictate every morsel you put in your mouth. But I don't know if this strategy of self-designed, self-monitored weight loss works very well. After all, the folks in that study were still overweight, even after an average of twenty years of attempted weight loss.

Researchers' question: What is the most satisfying feature of a weight-loss program?

Participants' response: In general, these folks were looking for noticeable or quick results.
My comment: Come on kids, wake up! Surely you've lived long enough to learn that the things in life that are worthwhile and lasting seldom come quickly. The effects of living the typical North American lifestyle for fifteen years will probably take fifteen years to reverse. And why are people in such a hurry? Are they anxious to get to the stage where "all" they have to do is maintain a healthy weight? Bad news: This stage isn't all that different from the stage where you're shedding pounds. Once you establish new, more healthful eating and exercise habits, you'll have to stick with them if you want to maintain a lean, fit body. Like my grandma always said, "It's about the journey, not the destination."

Researchers' question: Why is it hard to be successful in losing weight?

Participants' response: Many of the people surveyed said they weren't successful because it was difficult for them to make and maintain changes.
My comment: Most of the things that are worthwhile in life are difficult (and often time-consuming). But do we throw up our hands in despair and say it's just "too hard" to hold down a job, raise kids, or extend emotional support to family members and friends?

Participants' response: Another common excuse for failed weight-loss programs was not having enough time.
My comment: Spare me. Surely health and well-being are worth sacrificing an hour or two per day of watching TV, playing video games, complaining about being overweight, and making excuses. In case you forgot, you are in control of your schedule. Quit the pity party and put your time to better use.

Researchers' question: What are the barriers to weight-loss-treatment adherence?

Participants' response: Over 70 percent of those surveyed said they were unable to control what they ate when they were hungry.
My comment: This one's simple: If you don't surround yourself with crappy food, you won't be able to eat it. When you're hungry, it's good to eat. Keep healthful, natural, whole foods on hand, and when you're hungry, eat them. End of story.

Participants' response: Over 66 percent of the participants said they had difficulty staying motivated to eat appropriately.
My comment: Motivation is fickle. Set up a supportive environment, develop daily strategies, and build new, health-supporting habits. Start with baby steps and gradually build a new lifestyle. After all, you don't need motivation to keep on with business as usual.

Participants' response: Almost 60 percent of participants said their barriers to weight loss included using food as a reward.
My comment: Rewarding yourself is an excellent idea. Doing so with banana cream pie is not. Honestly, one of the best ways to ensure success in anything is to get the brain's reward system involved. Just be sure to choose health-supporting rewards. How about enjoying a walk in the park with someone you love, giving yourself some flowers, getting a massage—you get the idea. And in the end, isn't the best reward feeling better, being more fit, and enjoying a leaner body?

Participants' response: Another barrier to weight loss mentioned by many of those surveyed was being unable to resist tempting food.
My comment: Ah the allure of forbidden fruit! I discussed this in chapter 4, but in case you need a refresher, the answer here is simple (though it may seem heretical to those with a dieting mentality): Don't resist foods you enjoy. Don't put certain foods off-limits. When you put foods off-limits, you're more likely to have trouble resisting them. If you allow yourself to enjoy your favorite foods in reasonable amounts, you won't feel deprived and be inclined to binge.

Time to Kill

Americans watch about thirty-five hours of TV per week.[2] But you know what's really sad? The top two excuses I hear from people about why they don't eat nutritious foods and exercise is that they don't have enough money or time. If that sounds like your situation, I just may have a remedy. What if I said that one simple task could allow you to do all of the following:

- Have more money each month to spend on healthful food
- Have more time each month to prepare and enjoy healthful food and to exercise
- And, as a bonus, free yourself from annoying advertisements—particularly those that try to convince you to eat crappy food

Prepare to be amazed. My suggestion? Kill your TV. After all, what is TV, really, beyond an advertising vehicle with brief segments of entertainment interspersed between commercials that try to influence you to spend money or eat crappy food?

Putting the Life in "Lifestyle"

I learned something really neat in college: Lifestyle diseases are actually based on people's lifestyles. I think many people have lost sight of the fact that some simple lifestyle changes could drastically reduce their risk of "inevitable" or "mysterious" diseases like diabetes, heart disease, and cancer. Instead, they buy into the concept of "better living through modern chemistry": Why change your diet when you can take metformin (the first-line drug of choice for treating type 2 diabetes) and keep eating crap? Why cut out fatty animal products when you can take statins? Why confront difficult issues in life when you can take antidepressants? Why exercise to lower body fat and boost immune function when insurance companies will cover your chemo bills? (Okay, I admit that I put that last one in there to make you really think about why this isn't the greatest approach. If that didn't scare you, do not pass go, and do not collect two hundred dollars.)

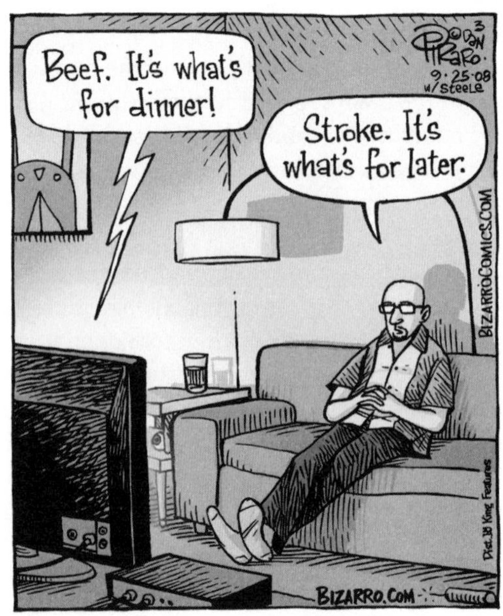

Beef. It's what's for dinner!
Stroke. It's what's for later.
DAN PIRARO 9·25·08 w/STEELE
BIZARROCOMICS.COM
BIZARRO.COM
Bizarro, reprinted by permission of Dan Piraro.

If you think "better living through modern chemistry" is preferable to changing your lifestyle, I have a few items for your consideration:

- **Long-term use of one diabetes drug increases heart attack risk by more than 40 percent.** An analysis of four studies involving more than fourteen thousand patients found that long-term use of the diabetes drug rosiglitazone (Avandia) increased the risk of heart attack by 42 percent and doubled the risk of heart failure.[3] Hmm, that makes it sound suspiciously like medications for a lifestyle-related disease can actually cause other diseases.
- **Spending on statin drugs went from $8 billion to almost $20 billion between 2000 and 2005.** In case you didn't know, statins are medications for high cholesterol (yes, a lifestyle-related condition). Thirty million people in the United States bought at least one statin drug in 2005—that was over 10 percent of Americans.[4] If you can't control your cholesterol levels with lifestyle changes, you aren't changing your lifestyle enough (except for the rare few with genetic disorders). Sorry, I know it may seem harsh,

but I had to say it. Hmm, so now you have one or more lifestyle-related diseases, not to mention mounting medical bills. That's enough to make anybody depressed.

- **Selective serotonin reuptake inhibitors (SSRIs), a group of drugs commonly used to treat depression, may double the risk of gastrointestinal bleeding.** When these drugs are taken with aspirin and other similar pain medications, the risk is more than 600 percent higher.[5] Hmm, so you're depressed because your health is in the toilet, and the antidepressants that supposedly help with that can actually cause *more* health problems? Yikes! Sounds like a vicious cycle to me.

What if you're fortunate enough that your only (current) major health issue is being fat? I still encourage you to just say no to drugs and to focus on diet and exercise instead. Sure, there are medications that might help with weight loss. But do you really think they're immune to issues with side effects? In case you're tempted, here are a few factoids for your consideration:

- Sibutramine (Meridia), an appetite suppressant formerly used to treat obesity, may cause heart attacks,[6] strokes, nausea, upset stomach, constipation, dizziness, headaches, joint or muscle pain, and, paradoxically, increased appetite. Folks, we have a winner! (Fortunately, sibutramine has been withdrawn from the market in most countries.)
- Orlistat (Alli), which prevents the absorption of fats and therefore is also used to treat obesity, may cause liver disease, not to mention fecal incontinence.[7] Nice!
- And how about exenatide (Byetta), used to treat type 2 diabetes? Turns out it may cause pancreatitis[8] and possibly thyroid cancer, not to mention diarrhea, nausea, and vomiting. Have fun with that!

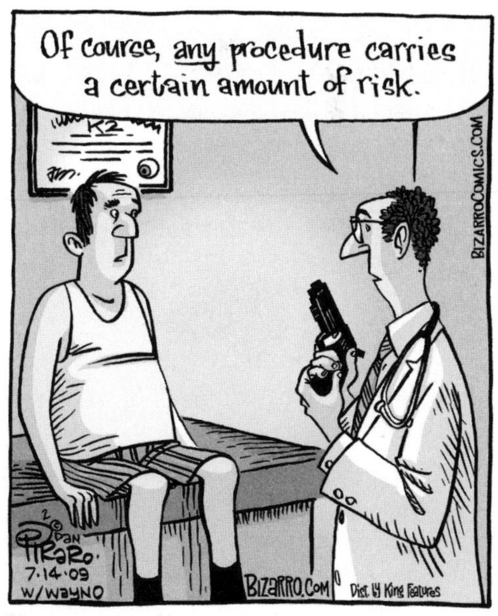

Bizarro, reprinted by permission of Dan Piraro.

I know it's hard to believe, but the human body doesn't always thrive on loads of synthetic pharmaceuticals.

Fortunately, there is an alternative: Adopting a lifestyle that decreases your risk of lifestyle-related diseases. If my credentials and all of the information outlined above aren't enough to convince you, then I suggest you take a page from Dean Ornish, MD, an expert in reversing heart disease through lifestyle changes. He says, "I don't understand why asking people to eat a well-balanced vegetarian diet is considered drastic, while it's medically conservative to cut people open or put them on powerful cholesterol-lowering drugs for the rest of their lives."[9]

Now or Later

Honestly, this isn't rocket science. We all know that in many areas of life it's best to attend to things along the way, rather than putting them off:

- If you don't maintain your house now, it will begin to fall apart and you'll have to devote a lot of time and money to major repairs later.
- If you don't balance your checkbook now, it will take a lot of time to figure out your finances later—and you may be looking at some hefty overdraft charges too.
- If you don't save money now, you'll have to work more later.
- If you don't put time and effort into your relationships now, you'll probably have to work double time at them later, if they last that long.
- If you don't file and pay your income taxes on time, you'll have to face a lot of penalties and interest later.
- If you don't work hard at your job now, you may have to find a new job later.
- If you don't clean up your lifestyle now, it's likely that your health will suffer later (if it isn't suffering already).

Some people think they can't find the time for preparing healthful food, exercising, getting enough sleep, and generally pursuing a more healthful lifestyle. These same people often seem to think they don't have the money for a gym membership, nutritious food, therapy, or working with a coach. (News flash: Eating less and eating at home more often might actually cost less, even in the short run.) But eventually, people who keep copping fattitudes will have to pay the piper. And in the long run, they'll probably lose a great deal of time to lifestyle diseases and spend a lot of money on doctors, diagnostic tests, treatments, surgery, and medications. And if those medications lead to new health complications? More time and money down the drain.

In the end, your health is up to you. Deal with it now or spend a lot of time and money on it later. It bears repeating: Take a look at what you do each day and realize that your schedule shows what you really care about. If you want to be fit and healthy, you must take time to prepare and eat nutritious food and get active on a regular basis.

Chapter 18

Fat People Get Overconfident with Their Weight-Management Skills

Constantly choosing the lesser of two evils is still choosing evil.

—Jerry Garcia

Sometimes I start feeling pretty high and mighty about my nutrition and exercise. Then I remember some of the humbling experiences over the years that helped me learn, once again, that one single decision can put me on the fast track to poor health and fitness and more body fat.

Decisions, Decisions

Think about it. Each of us has hundreds if not thousands of decisions to make every day, many of them related to health and body composition:

- What should I eat for breakfast?
- Should I exercise?
- Should I take my lunch to work today?
- Should I take the stairs?
- What beverages should I drink?
- Should I take a walking break?
- Should I park farther away from my destination?
- Should I walk my dog?
- Should I have salad or french fries?
- Do I really want that cookie?
- What time should I go to bed?
- Should I play smooth jazz to ensure a successful first date?

All of these decisions give us the opportunity to do something positive or negative. Each decision has consequences, affects our momentum, and may eventually lead to momentous changes (even the smooth jazz decision—trust me).

Most days of the week I make the decision to exercise shortly after I wake up. I've been making that decision fairly consistently for many years now. But each morning I'm only one decision away from moving in the wrong direction. I could easily hear the alarm, turn it off, and go back to sleep. That decision might prevent me from getting my daily exercise and, by virtue of the cascade effect, could have a negative impact not only on my fitness and maintaining a lean body, but also living according to my values and maintaining my self-esteem.

Here's another example: One day each week, I take time to shop and prepare food so that I have nutritious options on hand, ready to eat, throughout the week. This eliminates countless decisions about food. When mealtime rolls around, I just pull together a meal from fruits and veggies that I've washed and trimmed and precooked whole grains and beans. If I didn't have those items available, I would probably make different food choices.

Set yourself up for success by making some of your health-supporting decisions a routine way of life. Over time, these practices can become habitual and even mindless—in a good way. Honestly, deciding between oatmeal or a sausage biscuit for breakfast need not be a huge deal, on par with selecting a name for your firstborn. I'm living proof that making healthful food decisions on a daily basis does become easier with time. In my early teens, I was an honest-to-goodness junk food junkie. Now I wouldn't even consider stopping at a fast-food restaurant. That option just isn't on the list anymore. When you consistently make healthful decisions for long enough, it becomes what you do and who you are.

Think of some of the fittest and healthiest people you know. You have the same potential as they do. The difference is that they choose a healthful lifestyle, which translates into a lean and healthy body. To invoke an old truism, today really is the first day of the rest of your life. Heck, every minute brings you the opportunity to start again. Think of how liberating that is. In this moment, you can begin making decisions that will make you lean, healthy, and fit—and keep you that way.

Only Half the Battle

Most people who have struggled with being overweight know that losing weight is only half the battle. Actually, it's even less than that. The real challenge is *maintaining* weight loss. Sometimes I help clients achieve their weight-loss goals, only to see them return a few years later having regained all those pounds—and then some. What happens? People become cocky and complacent.

Being lean for life goes beyond eating reasonably sized meals, focusing on whole foods, saying no to fast food, and getting enough exercise. The fact is, it goes beyond any of the specific approaches recommended in this book. It involves your identity. If you manage to get fit, your new body won't be able to stay lean and healthy without the support of your heart, mind, and soul. The process of staying lean and healthy is a journey, and it's always evolving. Getting on that path may be arduous, but most folks are fairly motivated at first. Where you'll run into trouble is if you obsess about food, fitness, and weight loss for most of your waking hours.

Knowledge is only a small part of the success equation, and it isn't the limiting factor for most people. If I were to take fifty random people to the grocery store and ask them to point out five health-promoting foods, I imagine most of them could do it. Most people aren't boneheads. They know that leafy greens are more nutritious than fried pork rinds.

Having more knowledge beyond the basics doesn't necessarily ensure success. I know plenty of health professionals who make unhealthful choices about food and exercise every day. Lack of knowledge isn't the issue for them—and I bet it isn't for you, either (especially now that you've read most of this book). You don't need to know the details of human biochemistry or metabolism; you just need to know how to get nutritious food on your plate—and then you need to choose to do it (and choose to exercise).

In my view, losing weight is kind of like winning the lottery. It's fantastic! Or at least it is for a while. Unfortunately, many lottery winners wake up one day to find themselves no better off than they were before and wonder what the heck happened. The same is true of weight loss. Attitude—including lack of fattitudes—is the key to consolidating your gains (or in the case of weight, your losses). It's essential to transforming knowledge into a lifetime of good health and fitness. (For more on this, see *The Love-Powered Diet: Eating for Freedom, Health, and Joy*, by Victoria Moran).

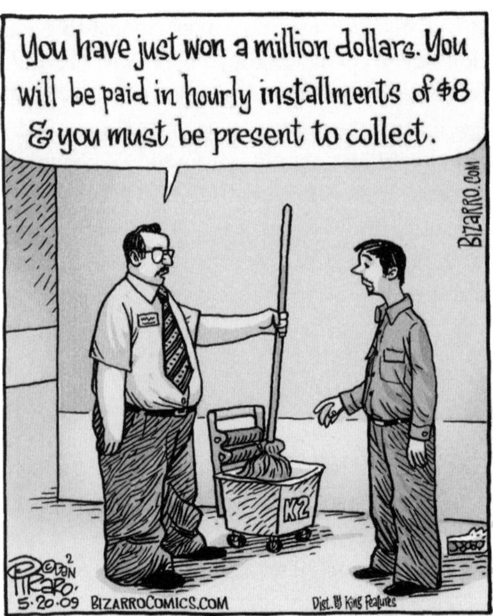

You have just won a million dollars. You will be paid in hourly installments of $8 & you must be present to collect.
BIZARRO.COM
K2
DAN PIRARO
5·20·09 BIZARROCOMICS.COM
Dist. By King Features
Bizarro, reprinted by permission of Dan Piraro.

Be Your Own Expert

How old are you right now? Why do I ask? Because I want you to consider that this is how many years of experience you have in nutrition, exercise, and, most importantly, your body. You have a wealth of knowledge; you just need to remember to tap into it—and to be honest with yourself when you examine your history and habits.

While you can gain knowledge and ideas from other people's approaches to nutrition, this can be a tricky proposition. A plan that works wonders for someone else may not work for you. In fact, it can be distracting and lead you down the wrong path. Instead, focus on knowledge that actually applies to you: Your years of eating experience, replete with trial and error, which equate to experimentation and feedback. You probably have a very good idea of which foods and habits make you feel lousy and lead to more body fat. If you're honest with yourself, you probably have an excellent idea about what's holding you back from your goals right now. I imagine that you know a lot more about what does and doesn't work for you than you give yourself credit for.

What type of things am I talking about? Well, since you're the expert on you, I can't be sure what does and doesn't work for you. But what I can share are some of the things that I've noticed are important for me:

- I listen to my body regarding both food and exercise. For example, I've noticed that I don't feel good after eating a lot of processed soy, so I eat black beans instead. I've noticed that my lower back aches when I do certain exercises, so I've found other ways to work those muscles.
- If I'm not hungry enough to eat real foods, like broccoli or lentils, I know I'm not really hungry.
- When I focus on how I feel after eating, rather than on how food will make me look, things go much better for me. The same goes for exercise.
- The all-or-none approach fails miserably for me when my incentives are weak or superficial. But when my incentives run deep, the all-or-none approach has been a useful tool. I've been able to use it successfully for major decisions, such as not drinking alcohol, using drugs, smoking, or eating animal products.
- Physical activity outside of the gym is critical for me to maintain a lean and fit body.
- Observing hunger cues trumps specific foods or meal scheduling. If I eat too much of anything, no matter what it is, or eat when I'm not really hungry I feel like crap and look the same.
- I can't read and eat. I can't watch TV and eat. I can't drive and eat. When I do, I don't listen to my body and I eat too much.
- Whenever my eating patterns take a turn for the worse, whether it's eating too much, eating too little, obsessing about food, or eating too much non-nutritious food, the actual issue is never food; rather, something in my life is out of balance but I'm ignoring it, and it's manifesting itself in my eating habits.
- To eat a healthful, plant-based diet each day, I need a purpose beyond how I look. Goals like bettering the planet, preventing animal suffering, and improving my long-term health give me powerful incentive.

You may find that some of these observations are spot-on for you. Others may not apply to you, or they may apply, but what works for you is different from what works for me. That's all fine. The goal is to notice your eating patterns and how they affect your weight and well-being, and then develop effective strategies. That's something you can only learn from years of personal experience, not from a textbook. So, what have you learned? What works for you? What doesn't? Here are a few questions to help you make the best use of your experience.

- How does your day go when you take the time for a nutritious breakfast? Do you have more sustained energy? Does it have any effect on your eating patterns for the rest of the day?
- Do you do better with the standard three meals a day, or with more frequent, smaller meals?
- Do you do well with strict diet rules and regulations? Do they lead you to long-term success, or do they eventually backfire?
- When you focus on nutritious food that tastes good and makes you feel good, does your desire for junk food and fast food tend to decline?
- How do different situations affect your eating habits? Do you tend to eat more moderately when you sit down for a meal with friends or family? How about when you prepare your own meals?
- Do you tend to overeat in certain situations, like while watching TV or using the Internet? Do you eat more or less around certain people?
- When you eat late at night, do you sleep well or poorly? Do you have more or less energy the next morning? Do specific food choices make a difference here?
- When you make the time to exercise, do you tend to feel more or less productive in other areas of life? How does regular exercise affect your self-esteem?
- If you use food to manage your moods or distract yourself from difficult life issues, how well does that strategy work for you in the long run? Does it make you feel better or worse about yourself and about life?

Big Fat Caveat

I love being exposed to views that oppose my own because it challenges what I believe and makes me question my approach. I constantly remind myself that I shouldn't get too comfortable with what I'm doing because nothing is 100 percent. Heck, even scientific research doesn't necessarily prove anything—in part because it can be so far removed from the complexities of real life. Before I went to Africa, I read a book that informed me I should play dead if I were charged by a hippo. Intellectually, this seemed to make sense. But once I arrived in Africa, the locals told me that if a hippo charged me I should run like hell and climb a tree if possible.

With many things in life, experience and practice are the best teachers. We learn that good strategies can fall short and that our beliefs or expectations kept us from trying better options.

As a dietitian and trainer, I want to offer you the best possible advice for improving your health and helping you get and stay lean. But I've got to be straight with you: things are always changing in the world of nutrition and fitness, and today's wisdom is often tomorrow's bad idea. So on behalf of myself and the dietetics community, I want to take a few minutes to apologize for some things we might have told you that weren't exactly accurate:

- All foods with fat are bad.
- Dieting is the best way to lose fat.
- Going to a gym is the only way to exercise.
- Dairy foods are great for bone health.
- "Fat-burning" supplements are useful.
- Whey protein is equivalent to holy water.
- Eating meat is necessary to get enough protein.
- Carbs make you fat.

Likewise, I'm sorry that we advised you to do the following:

- Eat six times per day, regardless of your hunger levels and eating preferences.
- Take a "cheat day" with eating.
- Replace sugar with artificial sweeteners.
- Count calories.
- Stop eating after 6:00 p.m.
- Think of all calories as being equal.
- Drink two quarts of water each day, no matter what.

Most importantly, I'm sorry for any information or advice in this book that won't make any sense in twenty years. Of course, learning new things can be exciting, but it can also be frustrating. Acquiring new knowledge means giving up previously held beliefs or, at a minimum, changing them. I'll be the first to apologize when something I say has been proven incorrect, but I'll never apologize for reversing my position, since that means I'm continuing to learn. I think we should all be willing to accept new ideas and consider new strategies. Don't be afraid to change what you believe.

Section IV:
The Fit Life

Chapter 19
Fit People (Surprise!) Think Like Fit People

The greatest discovery of my generation is that a human being can alter his life by altering his attitudes.

—William James

Think of something you've had success with. Maybe it was a job, hobby, or relationship, or maybe it was parenting, sports, or volunteering. Now think about the qualities you needed to attain that success. Seriously, list them out. I'll wait. . . .

What did you come up with? I bet your list included qualities like persistence, dedication, resilience, effort, planning, grit, honesty, integrity, humility, loyalty, organization, enthusiasm, and so forth. Imagine if you took those same qualities that have brought you success in other areas of life and applied them to eating, exercise, and health. What would happen?

If you've had success before—with anything—then you know what it takes to succeed, and you have the qualities required. Now it's just a matter of applying those qualities to shedding your fattitudes. In this chapter, I'll highlight the approaches I believe to be most powerful: eating real, whole foods; embracing new norms; courting temptation; and learning from the success of others.

Eat Real, Whole Foods

Our society sincerely needs a paradigm shift, especially regarding food. While some fat people know that their eating habits suck, many of them don't, and I can't always blame them. We're surrounded by 24/7 food marketing—typically for lowest-common-denominator foods, but also for "fabulous" new foodstuffs, purportedly all natural, that will enhance health and promote weight loss. If you buy that, just remember that the same company owns both Ben and Jerry's and Slim-Fast.

It boggles the mind that there are nearly twenty thousand new food products released each year. I don't think we need so many choices, especially when most of these new "foods" are nutritional losers. The foods we need to eat to be fit and healthy already exist. Most of them have been around for hundreds, if not thousands, of years. When you make eating real, whole foods a priority, you'll reap the benefits.

Need a little more motivation to adopt this key attitude? Just consider this Okinawan proverb: "One who eats whole food will be strong and healthy." Why should you care what the Okinawans say? Well, they enjoy extraordinary longevity, coupled with higher quality of life in their later years. They're typically lean and energetic, even in old age, and also have extremely low death rates from heart disease, cancer, and stroke—the top three killers in the United States.

At this point in the book you're probably well aware of why you should be eating real, whole foods, but here's a quick rundown: You'll stay healthier. You'll be leaner. Whole foods are more nutritious. Whole foods are more filling. Whole foods help regulate your appetite signals. It's more sustainable for the planet. And that's just for starters.

And I sincerely hope that at this point in the book you aren't wondering what the heck real, whole food actually is. But if you are, here are some simple ways to think about it: If a food wasn't around 150 years ago, it probably isn't real food. If it didn't come directly from a tree or plant and you can't make it in your own kitchen, it probably isn't real food. If it doesn't seem like real food, it probably isn't. If you're still confused, write this list on your forehead: vegetables, fruits, beans, grains, nuts, and seeds. To be fit, you need a foundation to build on, and that foundation is real food.

Embrace New Norms

By now you've undoubtedly developed a pretty good idea of what I consider to be a healthful lifestyle, and you assuredly know that I hold myself to that standard. Believe it or not, some people tell me that my health habits are extreme. In case the details of those health habits elude you, let's do a quick recap:

- I eat nutrient-dense, mostly organic whole foods.
- I eat a completely plant-based diet.
- I eat locally produced foods when possible.
- I don't eat fast food or any food that won't enhance my well-being.
- I challenge my body physically by exercising at least five hours per week, and I enjoy it.
- I sleep seven to nine hours each night and get up early.
- I don't drink alcohol.
- I don't use tobacco.
- I don't do drugs.
- I don't own a microwave.
- I don't have a car.

If that seems a little extreme, I'd argue it's simply because our social norms have become so skewed. One hundred years ago, much of that list probably would have applied to the average person. Maybe the best way to determine whether my lifestyle is extreme is to compare it to what has become normal in our culture:

- Relying on daily medications to treat preventable lifestyle diseases.
- Having to check blood sugar levels multiple times each day to avoid going into diabetic shock.
- Undergoing major heart surgery to fix vessels clogged by disease-promoting foods.
- Taking antidepressants and other mood-altering drugs because it's easier than facing difficult emotions and experiences.
- Not getting any exercise whatsoever most days of the week.
- Prioritizing TV over exercising, spending time outdoors, and eating nutritious foods.
- Wrecking one's health and endangering others' safety due to alcohol intoxication.
- Running out of clean water and land to feed and sustain future generations.

Which approach seems more extreme to you? The truth is, if you're "normal," you're fat and unhealthy. If you want to be lean and fit in these modern times, you need to embrace new norms. Why not join the "extreme and abnormal" club? After all, if enough folks do it, this will become the new social norm. You know that saying about "Be the change you want to see?" I'd definitely like to look around and see a nation of fit, happy, healthy people, and I bet you would too.

Courting Temptation

How do fit people do it? Year after year, they eat health-promoting food, exercise, get enough sleep, manage their stress, and maintain a lean body. I'd say it boils down to temptation. In our society, we're surrounded by negative temptations (aka junk food, fast food, alcohol, TV, and endless electronic devices) and encouragement to cave in to those temptations (aka advertisements). I say fight fire with fire. Surround yourself with tempting, healthful foods and give yourself free license to indulge in health-promoting activities. Let's take a look at how this might play out in real life.

If you eat the same healthful but bland foods over and over again, you'll get bored and may feel tempted by ready-to-eat junk food. But if you add spice to your meals by exploring a variety of recipes with new ingredients and flavors, that's a positive temptation.

If you keep unwashed vegetables shoved in the back of your fridge, you probably won't be tempted to eat them. But if you have containers filled with vegetables that are washed, cut, and ready to eat, that's a positive temptation.

If you think of basic food preparation tasks as boring, you may be tempted to eat out or eat prepared foods. But if you light a candle, put on some music, and think of cooking as a meditative process, that's a positive temptation.

If your workouts are tedious or boring, you'll probably be tempted not to do them. But if you focus on forms of exercise you enjoy, mix it up, and play some energizing upbeat tunes while you work out, that's a positive temptation.

If you exercise alone, you might get bored and feel tempted to skip your workouts. But if you have a workout partner to joke and compete with during a training session, that's a positive temptation.

Specific examples like these are all well and good, but to build positive temptation into a wide variety of areas of your unique life, you may benefit from some general guidelines. So, without further ado, here's my list of what makes something tempting:

- Tempting things are fun. This is the biggie. Figure out how to make things fun if you want to keep doing them.
- Tempting things appeal to our senses. They're enjoyable to watch, listen to, taste, smell, and feel.
- Tempting things often have a social component, like hanging out with friends or being part of a team.
- Tempting things make us feel good about ourselves. Achievements in the gym and with your eating habits should be innately rewarding, but you can help your progress along by giving yourself small tangible rewards for meaningful milestones.

Sometimes temptation is all about attitude. One of my top tips for keeping things fresh and fun is to pretend to be a kid again. Cast aside a stale exercise regimen and throw a Frisbee, pretend a monster is chasing you, or climb the monkey bars.

Here's one last tip about temptation, and it's a biggie: Things are usually tempting because they're in your face. Often they're convenient or easy. To remove unwanted temptations, flip that around. Make the stuff you don't want to do inconvenient or irritating. Don't buy cookies. If you leave them on the grocery shelf, you'll have to make another trip to get them—not too likely at 11 p.m. Instead, keep some apples close at hand, looking all nice and shiny. Discontinue your cable and put a bookshelf in front of your TV, then fill it up with plant-based cookbooks and some of the titles recommended in the Resources section. Keep your bike on the front porch, ready to use—or maybe even park it in front of your recliner.

Learn from the Success of Others

In this chapter I've emphasized the importance of eating whole foods, embracing new norms, and setting yourself up with positive temptations. You may be wondering if those approaches are sufficient for living a fit life. I honestly believe they are. However, most folks employ a wider variety of strategies to build a fit life. As discussed earlier in the book, you're the expert on you, and you'll need to figure out an approach that works for you.

Still, I've had the opportunity to work with thousands of people over the years, and I've learned a lot from them. Up to this point, I've shared a lot of the negatives: what I've learned about fattitudes and why they're a recipe for disaster. Now it's time to turn the tables and look at some of the best tips I've learned from colleagues and clients. These come straight from people who are getting it done, living—and thinking—like fit people.

- **Don't drink calories.** This is a big one. Simply limiting beverages to water, tea, and coffee would probably be enough for many people to lose some (or a lot of) fat without doing anything else.
- **Balance your fat intake.** Healthful fats play an important role in a well-rounded diet, so don't try to avoid them. Instead, favor monounsaturated fats and omega-3s. Good sources include almonds, avocados, chia seeds, coconut, edamame, flaxseeds, hempseeds, macadamia nuts, olives, tempeh, and walnuts.
- **Don't eat low-fat, low-carb, reduced-calorie, sugar-free, or diet packaged foods.** That's just poor-quality food masquerading as something healthful. Eat real, whole, nutritious foods. If you want something sweet, eat fruit. If you want something rich, eat an avocado or a handful of nuts.
- **Be open to new foods.** Understand that the more you eat nutritious foods, the more you'll want them. (And, not surprisingly, the same goes for unhealthful foods, so try to avoid them completely or limit them substantially).
- **Don't plan for "cheat meals."** Occasionally, you'll eat some crummy food or overeat. We all do. Since you're going to do it anyway, there's certainly no need to include it in your schedule. (And don't forget, your schedule says volumes about what you care about.)
- **Eat when you're hungry.** If you eat regularly and listen to your genuine hunger cues, you'll probably feel more satisfied, stabilize your blood sugar, have increased and sustained energy, and improve your performance in exercise—oh, and drop a fair amount of body fat too. Your body will tell you whether that means six small meals per day, three moderate meals, or something in between.
- **Maintain a low A or high B average.** Scoring 80 to 90 percent was good enough to get your driver's license, and it's also good enough for nutrition. Don't try to be perfect. Just do the smart thing a majority of the time, forever.

- **Stop (or don't start) the cycle of dieting.** Diets don't work; trust me. In my profession, I see this time and again. I can assure you that the people who are most zealous about diets are the same folks who are the most overweight. Remember, healthful nutrition and regular exercise are a lifestyle, not a temporary program.
- **Recognize and understand your unhealthful eating patterns.** Once you learn to recognize when you're eating to soothe your emotions, you can begin to change this behavior. Emotions aren't right or wrong; they just are, and if you learn to accept them and sit with them, they will eventually recede and give way to other emotions. This concept is simple, but living by it can be hard, so work with a professional if need be.
- **Exercise four to seven hours per week.** Build in some regular exercise—just promise me that you'll find physical activities that you enjoy doing so you'll stick with it. Don't expect exercise to happen unless you prioritize it.
- **Be realistic.** You may think it would be fun to look like Mr. or Ms. America, but your ideal weight is the one at which you're doing the most you're willing to do to keep it there. With that approach, you'll wind up having a body you can live with, at that perfect balance point between what's mentally tolerable and what's physically sustainable.
- **Take ownership of yourself—body, mind, life, and spirit.** This tip isn't about blame; it's about responsibility. It also isn't about fairness; it's about accountability and accepting the consequences of your actions. Don't view this as a gloomy or overwhelming prospect. When you fully appreciate how much power you have over your life, it's incredibly empowering.
- **Attitude reigns supreme.** You will never succeed if you think you can't. You need to be on board with what you're doing, 100 percent. Sure, there will be tough times. Short-circuit them by learning how to enjoy the process of becoming lean and fit—because if you're miserable along the way, you definitely won't succeed.
- **Practice gratitude.** Take a few minutes each morning to write down or think about everything that you're thankful for. This can have a profound effect on well-being.

And now for a bonus tip. Since I just gave you a list of rules that have brought other people success this one may seem kind of ironic, but here goes: Don't follow anyone else's rules. Seriously, don't follow anyone else's rules (including those in this book) unless they work for you and enrich your journey through life. People tend to get wrapped up in diet tips and guidelines, but most of them are worthless. If an approach sounds good to you, try it. If it doesn't, don't try it. If you do try it, be sure to honestly assess how it's working for you. This applies to all areas of life: keep evaluating, experimenting, and evolving.

The Bottom Line

Okay, you've stuck with me through almost the entire book. I wish I were there in person so I could give you your gold star. Instead, I'll give you the bottom line. Are you ready? Brace yourself! There is no bottom line.

I know it feels great to latch on to a straightforward, clear-cut solution or approach, but folks, that isn't how life works, and it's definitely not how good health works. There are simply too many variables involved in fitness and body weight. What I can give you is what you've encountered throughout this book: information that will raise your awareness about eating, exercise, and body fat. Having this awareness is the first step in making meaningful changes. Now it's up to you. Only you can decide to evaluate the choices you make each day.

As you implement what you've learned here, try to focus on behaviors rather than outcomes. After all, behaviors set the stage for outcomes. Plus, behaviors are more easily controlled than outcomes. Focus on who you want to be and how you want to feel—and perhaps most importantly, have fun with it. That's a huge part of a healthy attitude. If you've learned anything from this book, hopefully it's that healthy attitudes create healthy people, and healthy people have healthy bodies.

Still, you may be the type of person who longs for a little structure in life, and there's no crime in that. If you're disappointed that there's no bottom line, perhaps you'll find some solace in the next (and final) chapter, where I outline a simple plan for transforming your diet, your lifestyle, and your body.

Chapter 20
My Simple Plan to Get Lean, Stay Lean, Prevent Disease, and Feel Amazing

Eighty percent of success is showing up.
—Woody Allen

Maybe you've seen the TV show *30 Days*, a reality show created by Morgan Spurlock (the genius behind the film *Super Size Me*). The basic premise is having people immerse themselves in a different life for thirty days to see how they're affected. This might mean working for minimum wage, being in prison, or living off the grid.

Without fail, the experience is enlightening. Do the people on *30 Days* always convert to a new way of thinking or living? Heck no. However, living in someone else's shoes for thirty days certainly changes their perspectives and helps them understand different ways of living.

So, why are we talking about TV when you know by now that I'm mostly against it? In case you hadn't guessed, my challenge to you is to live like a fit person for thirty days. Let the concepts in this book guide your daily decisions about food, exercise, and attitudes. Just give it a go and see what happens.

A Simple Plan

I believe that dropping the fattitudes and making good decisions about small things, day in, day out, can turn anyone's life around. But as I acknowledged at the end of the previous chapter, some folks do thrive on structure and guidelines. As coach Mike Krzyzewski says in his book *Leading with the Heart*, "The truth is that many people set rules to keep from making decisions."[1] And you know what? That's okay.

So if you're a person who doesn't do well with choices and prefer to have a plan laid out for you—voilà!—here's a seven-week plan for getting lean, staying that way, preventing disease, and generally feeling amazing. What's not to like about that?

Week 1

- Eat plenty of vegetables each day. They can be fresh, frozen, canned, or from a salad bar; the source doesn't matter.
- Do about one hour of your favorite exercise, spread out over the week. That's less than nine minutes a day, so don't cop the fattitude that you don't have the time or energy.

Week 2

- Eat plenty of vegetables each day
- Eat plenty of fruit each day. Again, it can be fresh, frozen, canned, or pulled from your neighbor's apple tree.
- Do about one and a half hours of your favorite exercise over the course of the week. No whining: That's less than thirteen minutes a day.

Week 3

- Eat plenty of vegetables each day.
- Eat plenty of fruit each day.
- Eat some beans each day. They can be in the form of baked beans, beans and rice, bean soup, chili, edamame, falafel, hummus, or a bean burger, bean burrito, or bean salad.
- Do about two hours of your favorite exercise. No complaining: That's barely seventeen minutes per day.

Week 4

- Eat plenty of vegetables each day.
- Eat plenty of fruit each day.
- Eat some beans each day.
- Eat some nuts and seeds each day. Almonds, cashews, hazelnuts, peanuts, pecans, pistachios, walnuts, chia seeds, flaxseeds, hempseeds, pumpkin seeds, sunflower seeds, almond butter, cashew butter, peanut butter—all are delicious, and I'm sure you won't have any trouble working them into your diet.
- Do about two and a half hours of your favorite exercise. For you math degenerates, that's less than twenty-two minutes per day.

Week 5

- Eat plenty of vegetables each day.
- Eat plenty of fruit each day.
- Eat some beans each day.
- Eat some nuts and seeds each day.
- Eat some whole grains each day. Here, I'm talking literally whole grains, cooked or sprouted: amaranth, barley, brown rice, buckwheat, corn, Kamut, millet, oats, quinoa, wild rice, and so forth.
- Do about three hours of your favorite exercise this week. That's just over twenty-five minutes a day.

Week 6

- Eat plenty of vegetables each day.
- Eat plenty of fruit each day.
- Eat some beans each day.
- Eat some nuts and seeds each day.
- Eat some whole grains each day.
- Drink some green tea each day. Get some tea leaves or tea bags and brew your own tea. Avoid the bottled stuff unless it's your only option.
- Do about three and a half hours of your favorite exercise. That averages out to half an hour per day. At this point, you should be starting to feel great about being more buff!

Week 7

- Eat plenty of vegetables each day.
- Eat plenty of fruit each day.
- Eat some beans each day.
- Eat some nuts and seeds each day.
- Eat some whole grains each day.
- Drink some green tea each day.
- Do around four hours of your favorite exercise.
- Try a new food this week. From arugula to golden zucchini and from kumquats to loquats to mangoes, there's a delicious world of fruits and vegetables out there. Experiment and discover what you like. Extend this same approach to beans, grains, nuts, seeds, and even beverages, such as various herbal teas.

Week 8 and Beyond

- Continue to follow the dietary guidelines from week 7 (including experimenting with new foods).
- Take a vitamin B_{12} supplement on a regular basis. While supplementing with vitamin B_{12} is important for everyone, regardless of their dietary choices, it is especially important for people eating a highly plant-based diet.
- Aim for five hours of total exercise time each week. That's less than forty-five minutes daily.
- Aim for seven to nine hours of restful sleep each night.
- Go on a media diet: Watch less TV, read fewer popular magazines, and limit your Internet time. And above all, be wary, very wary, of crappy popularized advice regarding nutrition and exercise.
- Get outside and enjoy some fresh air for twenty to thirty minutes each day. As a bonus, sunshine will help your body produce vitamin D.
- Give yourself an enjoyable reward, like a massage, an easy yoga class, a dry sauna, or time in the Jacuzzi. You deserve it!

Parting Pep Talk

Did you notice anything about this plan? It's all about what you *can* do, not about what you shouldn't do or what you should give up. It's about setting yourself up for success by focusing on foods and lifestyle habits that are good for you. Give it a try! What do you have to lose? (Other than a few pounds, that is.)

Honestly, aren't your health and well-being worth a seven-week experiment? While I can't guarantee that you'll stick to these suggestions or that they will be everything you ever dreamed of in terms of weight loss, I can guarantee one thing: It will definitely help you shed some fattitudes, and that's a huge step in the right direction.

If you need help or more motivation along the way, check out the books and DVDs listed in the Resources section. You can find more resources at precisionnutrition.com, and on my blogs at precisionnutrition.com/category/blog and precisionnutrition.com/category/articles. And if you find you just can't do it on your own, consider working with a fitness professional. Remember, your body and your health are on the line. You deserve to succeed, and you need to set yourself up for success.

Resources

I'll own it. I'm an information junkie. As a dietitian and trainer, I've read a vast multitude of health-related books. While I can't pull that spoon of ice cream out of your mouth or force you to get up out of your recliner and do something active, I can give you the benefit of my experience and guide you toward some of the books and other resources that I've found most helpful and compelling. Some of them will give you more knowledge and strategies for getting lean and staying that way—and changing your fattitudes. All of them will inspire you and change your life.

Books

Breaking Out of Food Jail: How to Free Yourself from Diets and Problem Eating, Once and for All, by Jean Antonello
Written by a nutritionist and nurse, this book examines the ugly truth behind dieting: losing weight through excessive restriction involves famine, which eventually leads to feasting, creating a vicious cycle. Her "radical" solution is to eat when you're hungry and stop when you're full.

Breaking the Food Seduction: The Hidden Reasons Behind Food Cravings—and Seven Steps to End Them, by Neal Barnard
Food isn't ever addictive. And yes, Virginia, there is a Santa Claus. . . . Written by the founder of the Physicians Committee for Responsible Medicine, this book discusses the addictive properties of food and how to free yourself from cravings. It also includes numerous recipes to help you rehabilitate your diet.

The Beck Diet Solution: Train Your Brain to Think Like a Thin Person, by Judith Beck
For all of the cognitive behavioral junkies out there (hello California!), this book has it all. The basic premise is that thinking and eating like a thin person can be learned—just like learning to drive. If I may be so bold as to say it, I believe this book offers techniques that will serve as the foundation of weight-management treatment in the future.

The Metabolism Advantage: An Eight-Week Program to Rev Up Your Body's Fat-Burning Machine, by John Berardi
If you recall that I work with John Berardi at a company called Precision Nutrition, you just might think this recommendation is biased. You caught me. But I work at Precision Nutrition because I truly believe in their approach, and not just in the world of nutrition. This offering from John Berardi shatters the myth that age-related weight gain is inevitable. It includes information on diet, exercise, and supplements that will help you burn calories and build muscle.

The Precision Nutrition System, by John Berardi
If you're frustrated with diets and want some guidance in figuring out what nutritional strategy will work for you, pick up *The Precision Nutrition System*, which includes nutrition guidebooks, the cookbook *Gourmet Nutrition*, and goal-specific exercise programs.

The Incredible Shrinking Critic: Seventy-Five Pounds and Counting—My Excellent Adventure in Weight Loss, by Jami Bernard
To be honest, the title of this book made me feel a little skeptical. Then I read it and developed and a new outlook on maintaining weight loss. Enough said.

The Blue Zones: Lessons for Living Longer from the People Who've Lived the Longest, by Dan Buettner
This book goes way beyond looking good in a tank top. The author examined four communities in California, Japan, Italy, and Costa Rica renowned for longevity and then, with the help of epidemiologists and other scientists, identified nine factors contributing to longer life. Brace yourself for the big news: avoiding processed food and exercising more are two of the factors.

Your Body Revival: Weight Loss Straight Talk, by Dave Draper
Written by a former Mr. America, Mr. World, and Mr. Universe, this book is a compendium of solid, no-nonsense information about weight loss and training. If you have even a remote interest in bodybuilding—and even if you don't—you will enjoy this book. And if Dave Draper can't inspire and motivate you, no one can.

Eating Animals, by Jonathan Safran Foer
This is an excellent book about the standard American diet (no surprise that the acronym for that is SAD). After learning his wife was pregnant, Jonathan Foer wanted to settle his own dietary debate about vegetarianism once and for all, so he'd be sure of the best diet for his child. If you're still attached to eating meat, his exposé of factory farms will probably help you pry that greasy burger out of your hands.

Skinny Bitch: A No-Nonsense Tough-Love Guide for Savvy Girls Who Want to Stop Eating Crap and Start Looking Fabulous and *Skinny Bastard: A Kick-in-the-Ass for Real Men Who Want to Stop Being Fat and Start Getting Buff*, by Rory Freedman and Kim Barnouin
Talk about irreverent! If you want to read something that will help you eat better while also making you laugh until your abdominals cramp, look no further.

Quantum Wellness: A Practical and Spiritual Guide to Health and Happiness, by Kathy Freston
Brace yourself, folks: There's more to wellness than eating and exercise. When was the last time you helped others or did some meditation? This book challenges a lot of assumptions about weight loss and health and suggests that the answer lies in focusing not just on the body, but also on the mind and spirit.

Eat for Health: Lose Weight, Keep It Off, Look Younger, Live Longer, by Joel Fuhrman
The author of this two-book set is a physician who specializes in using nutritional and natural approaches to prevent and reverse disease. One volume covers the mental makeover, and the other covers the body makeover. This set is full of great ideas on simple eating strategies, along with plenty of recipes.

The End of Overeating: Taking Control of the Insatiable American Appetite, by David Kessler
David Kessler, MD, got his medical degree from Harvard, and then for good measure he got a law degree. He's also a former FDA commissioner who heroically tackled the tobacco industry. Given those credentials, it's eye-opening that he views food addiction as the number one public health issue in the United States. In this book, he examines how food manufacturers have cracked the code of food addictions and used that information to create a nation of food junkies.

The Pleasure Trap: Mastering the Hidden Force That Undermines Health and Happiness, by Douglas J. Lisle and Alan Goldhammer
These authors offer the liberating insight that food issues may reflect a biological challenge, rather than a character flaw. Alas, insight may not be enough to help you put down that double-bacon cheeseburger. Fortunately, this book also provides solid advice on specific behavioral steps for escaping the pleasure trap.

Eat What You Love, Love What You Eat: How to Break Your Eat-Repent-Repeat Cycle, by Michelle May
Still scarfing down meals without a second thought? This book can help. What's not to like about an approach that involves *not* being afraid of food?

Fat, Broke, and Lonely No More: Your Personal Solution to Overeating, Overspending, and Looking for Love in All the Wrong Places, by Victoria Moran
Anyone who follows my articles and blogs knows that I'm a huge fan of Victoria Moran, and this is one of my favorite books of all time. Laugh now, but call me in two years after you've done a U-turn and left your negative habits in the dust.

Fit From Within: 101 Simple Secrets to Change Your Body and Your Life—Starting Today and Lasting Forever, by Victoria Moran
This book changed my life (in a *good* way). And if you doubt Victoria Moran's credentials, consider this: After decades of struggling with weight, she finally found an approach that helped her shed an extra 60 pounds—for good. Her secret? Self-acceptance, self-nurturing, and spirituality. Among her 101 simple secrets, I'm sure you'll find more than a few that are effective for you.

The Love-Powered Diet: Eating for Freedom, Health, and Joy, by Victoria Moran
What can I say? Victoria Moran has had an enormous impact on my life and eating habits, personally and professionally. This particular book earned gold stars from Rory Freedman (author of *Skinny Bitch*), John Robbins (vegan advocate extraordinaire), and Dean Ornish, MD (an expert in reversing heart disease through lifestyle changes).

Strength for Life: The Fitness Plan for the Rest of Your Life, by Shawn Phillips
Exercise is great; focused training is even better. This book on strength training offers a twelve-week program that can transform your body, and quite possibly sharpen your mind and energize your life along the way.

In Defense of Food: An Eater's Manifesto, by Michael Pollan
This is one of my favorite books exploring the topic of nutrition. The author's bottom line? "Eat food. Not too much. Mostly plants." (Hey, maybe *that's* the one weird, simple, old trick all of those Internet ads hint at!)

Appetite for Profit: How the Food Industry Undermines Our Health and How to Fight Back, by Michele Simon
If I haven't convinced you that the food industry is twisted, read this book by a public health policy expert and professor of law. You just might get so mad that you'll boycott those chicken tenders.

Intuitive Eating, by Evelyn Tribole and Elyse Resch
After reading *Eat What You Love, Love What You Eat*, by Michelle May, are you *still* scarfing down meals without a second thought? Maybe this book will get the point across: although it may seem counterintuitive, if you make peace with food and rediscover the pleasures of eating, you stand a better chance of overcoming compulsive eating and other food issues.

Hungry: Lessons Learned on the Journey from Fat to Thin, by Allen Zadoff
If you're a compulsive eater, buy this book and set up a shrine for it. You may think your struggle with weigh is unique—until you read many of your own thoughts committed to the written page by Zadoff. You'll find encouragement in the author's success story, and inspiration in how the journey transformed his life.

DVDs

Killer at Large, by Steven Greenstreet

A film about obesity featuring Bill Clinton, Arnold Schwarzenegger, Michael Pollan, and Ralph Nader? That's what I call entertainment value *plus* excellent information on the obesity epidemic and possible solutions. For more information, check out the movie's website: killeratlarge.com.

Food, Inc., by Robert Kenner

A hard-hitting exposé of the U.S. food industry, addressing a wide range of issues from diabetes, obesity, and foodborne illness to environmental impacts and the global food crisis to the corporate profiteering and the downsides of valuing convenience over environmental impact to the horrors of factory farming to . . . If I weren't getting breathless I could go on and on about how important this film is. But seeing is believing, so just go watch it. To learn more, check out the film's website: foodincmovie.com.

Earthlings, directed by Shaun Monson

Earthlings is one of the best films I've ever seen. In about two hours this movie will bring you up to speed on how animals are being treated. But I have to warn you. After watching it you may want to find your favorite blanket, crawl into your closet, and rock back and forth, shuddering and cursing our species for the way we treat our fellow beings on this planet. To get started, check out the movie's website: earthlings.com

References

Introduction

1. Beers, Mark H., and Robert Berkow (eds.). 1999. *The Merck Manual of Diagnosis and Therapy*, 17th edition, section 1, chapter 5, page 60. West Point, PA: Merck Research Laboratories.

2. Li, Choyang, et al. 2009. "Estimates of body composition with dual-energy X-ray absorptiometry in adults." *American Journal of Clinical Nutrition* 90(6):1457–1465.

3. Pilon, Brad. 2009. "Body fat—When average isn't good enough." Accessed August 21, 2010. bradpilon.com/weight-loss/body-fat-when-average-isnt-good-enough.

4. Water Footprint Network. 2010. "Product water footprints: Animal products." Accessed August 21, 2010. waterfootprint.org/?page=files/Animal-products.

5. Imhoff, Daniel. 2010. *The CAFO Reader: The Tragedy of Industrial Animal Factories.* Healdsburg, CA: Watershed Media.

6. Food and Agriculture Organization of the United Nations. 2009. "1.02 billion people hungry." Accessed August 20, 2010. www.fao.org/news/story/en/item/20568/icode.

7. Worldwatch Institute. 2004. "Now, it's not personal! But like it or not, meat-eating is becoming a problem for everyone on the planet." *World Watch* 17(4):13.

8. USDA Agricultural Projections to 2016. Last updated February 14, 2007. ers.usda.gov/publications/oce071/.

9. The Daily Beast. 2011. "Alien invasion!" *Newsweek*, July 7, 1996. Accessed August 14, 2011. thedailybeast.com/newsweek/1996/07/07/alien-invasion.html.

10. Vegetarian Resource Group. 2009. "How many vegetarians are there?" Accessed August 20, 2010. vrg.org/press/2009poll.htm.

11. Vegetarian Resource Group. 1997. "How many vegetarians are there?" Accessed August 20, 2010. vrg.org/journal/vj97sep/979poll.htm.

12. Worm, Boris, et al. 2006. "Impacts of biodiversity loss on ocean ecosystem services." *Science* 314(5800):787–790.

13. Stuart, Tristan. 2009. *Waste: Uncovering the Global Food Scandal.* New York: Norton.

14. Hall, Kevin D., et al. 2009. "The progressive increase of food waste in America and its environmental impact." *PLoS One* 4(11):e7940.

15. Hellmich, Nanci. 2009. "Obesity a key link to soaring health tab as costs double." *USA Today*, July 7. Accessed August 21, 2010. usatoday.com/news/health/2009-07-27-costofobesity_N.htm.

16. Centers for Disease Control and Prevention. 2009. "Cigarette smoking among adults and trends in smoking cessation—United States, 2008." *Morbidity and Mortality Weekly Report* 58(44):1227–1232.

17. Weingarten, Hemi. 2010. "Dieting trumps sex, career, and TV. Really?" *Fooducate* (blog). Accessed August 21, 2010. fooducate.com/blog/2010/08/18/dieting-trumps-sex-career-and-tv-really.

18. Sharma, Robin. 2006. *The Greatness Guide: Powerful Secrets for Getting to World Class*, pages 64–65. New York: Harperbusiness.

Chapter 1

1. Siega-Riz, Anna M., Barry M. Popkin, and Terri Carson. 1998. "Trends in breakfast consumption for children in the United States from 1965–1991." *American Journal of Clinical Nutrition* 67(4 suppl):748S–756S.

2. Greenwood, Jessica L. J., and Joseph B. Stanford. 2008. "Preventing or improving obesity by addressing specific eating patterns." *Journal of the American Board of Family Medicine* 21(2):135–140.

3. Cho, Sungsoo, et al. 2003. "The effect of breakfast type on total daily energy intake and body mass index: results from the Third National Health and Nutrition Examination Survey (NHANES III)." *Journal of the American College of Nutrition* 22(4):296–302.

4. Kant, Ashima K., et al. 2008. "Association of breakfast energy density with diet quality and body mass index in American adults: National Health and Nutrition Examination Surveys, 1999–2004." *American Journal of Clinical Nutrition* 88(5):1396–1404.

5. Mui, Ylan Q. 2010. "Fast-food breakfast sales decline as fewer head to work." *Washington Post*, February 21. Accessed August 21, 2010. washingtonpost.com/wp-dyn/content/article/2010/02/20/AR2010022003718.html.

6. Pearson, Natalie, Stuart J. H. Biddle, and Trish Gorely. 2009. "Family correlates of breakfast consumption among children and adolescents: A systematic review." *Appetite* 52(1):1–7.

7. Lundgren, Jennifer D., et al. 2008. "A descriptive study of non-obese persons with night eating syndrome and a weight-matched comparison group." *Eating Behaviors* 9(3):343–351.

8. Yunsheng, Ma, et al. 2003. "Association between eating patterns and obesity in a free-living US adult population." *American Journal of Epidemiology* 158(1):85–92.

9. Timlin, Maureen T., et al. 2008. "Breakfast eating and weight change in a 5-year prospective analysis of adolescents: Project EAT (Eating Among Teens)." *Pediatrics* 121(3):e638–e645.

10. De Castro, John M. 2007. "The time of day and the proportions of macronutrients eaten are related to total daily food intake." *British Journal of Nutrition* 98(5):1077–1083.

11. De Castro, John M. 2004. "The time of day of food intake influences overall intake in humans." *Journal of Nutrition* 134(1):104–111.

Chapter 2

1. Sierra-Johnson, Justo, et al. 2008. "Eating meals irregularly: A novel environmental risk factor for the metabolic syndrome." *Obesity* (Silver Spring) 16(6):1302–1307.

2. Otsuka, Rei, et al. 2006. "Eating fast leads to obesity: Findings based on self-administered questionnaires among middle-aged Japanese men and women." *Journal of Epidemiology* 16(3):117–124.

3. Maruyama, Koutatsu, et al. 2008. "The joint impact on being overweight of self-reported behaviours of eating quickly and eating until full: Cross-sectional survey." *British Medical Journal* 337:a2002.

4. Batterham, Rachel L., et al. 2002. "Gut hormone PYY(3-36) physiologically inhibits food intake." *Nature* 418(6898):650–654.

5. Scherwitz, Larry, and Deborah Kesten. 2005. "Seven eating styles linked to overeating, overweight, and obesity." *Explore* (NY) 1(5):342–359.

6. Stroebele, Nanette, and John M. De Castro. 2004. "Effect of ambience on food intake and food choice." *Nutrition* 20(9):821–838.

7. Liebman, Michael, et al. 2003. "Dietary intake, eating behavior, and physical activity–related determinants of high body mass index in rural communities in Wyoming, Montana, and Idaho." *International Journal of Obesity and Related Metabolic Disorders* 27(6):684–692.

8. Blass, Elliott M., et al. 2006. "On the road to obesity: Television viewing increases intake of high-density foods." *Physiology and Behavior* 88(4–5):597–604.

9. Moran, Victoria. 1997. *Shelter for the Spirit: How to Make Your Home a Haven in a Hectic World*, page 7. New York: HarperCollins.

Chapter 3

1. Berthoud, Hans-Rudolf. 2002. "Multiple neural systems controlling food intake and body weight." *Neuroscience and Biobehavioral Reviews* 26(4):393–428.

2. Khan, Kim. 2010. "How does your debt compare?" *MSN Money*. Accessed August 21, 2010. moneycentral.msn.com/content/savinganddebt/p70581. asp (expired).

3. Trivedi, Bijal P. 2010. "The agony and the ecstasy of the calorie." In *What I Eat: Around the World in Eighty Diets*, pages 120–121. Napa, CA: Material World Books.

Chapter 4

1. Stice, Eric, Katherine Presnell, and Heather Shaw. 2005. "Psychological and behavioral risk factors for obesity onset in adolescent girls: A prospective study." *Journal of Consulting and Clinical Psychology* 73(2):195–202.

2. Shunk, Jennifer A., and Leann L. Birch. 2004. "Girls at risk for overweight at age 5 are at risk for dietary restraint, disinhibited overeating, weight concerns, and greater weight gain from 5 to 9 years." *Journal of the American Dietetic Association* 104(7):1120–1126.

3. Tanofsky-Kraff, Marian, et al. 2006. "A prospective study of psychological predictors of body fat gain among children at high risk for adult obesity." *Pediatrics* 117(4):1203–1209.

4. Neumark-Sztainer, Diane, et al. 2007. "Why does dieting predict weight gain in adolescents? Findings from project EAT-II: A 5-year longitudinal study." *Journal of the American Dietetic Association* 107(3):448–455.

Chapter 5

1. Taub-Dix, Bonnie. 2010. *Read It Before You Eat It: How to Decode Food Labels and Make the Healthiest Choice Every Time.* New York: Plume.

2. U.S. Department of Agriculture Economic Research Service. 2007. "The U.S. grain consumption landscape: Who eats grain, in what form, where, and how much." *ERS Report Summary*, November. Accessed August 22, 2010. ers.usda.gov/publications/err50/err50_reportsummary.pdf.

3. Anderson, James W., et al. 2009. "Health benefits of dietary fiber." *Nutrition Reviews* 67(4):188–205.

4. Higgins, Peter, and John F. Johanson. 2004. "Epidemiology of constipation in North America: A systematic review." *American Journal of Gastroenterology* 99(4):750–759.

5. Sanjoaquin, Miguel A., et al. 2004. "Nutrition and lifestyle in relation to bowel movement frequency: A cross-sectional study of 20630 men and women in EPIC-Oxford." *Public Health Nutrition* 7(1):77.

6. Bandyopadhyay, Atrayee, Sarbani Ghoshal, and Anita Mukherjee. 2008. "Genotoxicity testing of low-calorie sweeteners: Aspartame, acesulfame-K, and saccharin." *Drug and Chemical Toxicology* 31(4):447–457.

7. Whitehouse, Christina R., Joseph Boullata, and Linda A. McCauley. 2008. "The potential toxicity of artificial sweeteners." *AAOHN Journal* 56(6):251–259.

8. Nettleton, Jennifer A., et al. 2009. "Diet soda intake and risk of incident metabolic syndrome and type 2 diabetes in the Multi-Ethnic Study of Atherosclerosis (MESA)." *Diabetes Care* 32(4):688–694.

9. Ludwig, David S. 2009. "Artificially sweetened beverages: Cause for concern." *Journal of the American Medical Association* 302(22):2477–2478

Chapter 6

1. Rolls, Barbara J., et al. 1998. "Volume of food consumed affects satiety in men." *American Journal of Clinical Nutrition* 67(6):1170–1177.

2. Ello-Martin, Julia A., Jenny H. Ledikwe, and Barbara J. Rolls. 2005. "The influence of food portion size and energy density on energy intake: Implications for weight management." *American Journal of Clinical Nutrition* 82(1 suppl):236S–241S.

3. Rolls, Barbara J., and Robert A. Barnett. 2000. *The Volumetrics Weight-Control Plan: Feel Full on Fewer Calories*, page 19. New York: Harper Paperbacks.

4. Anderson, James W., et al. 2009. "Health benefits of dietary fiber." *Nutrition Reviews* 67(4):188–205.

Chapter 7

1. International Food Information Council Foundation. 2010. *2010 Food and Health Survey: Consumer Attitudes toward Food Safety, Nutrition, and Health*. Accessed July 18, 2011. foodinsight.org/Resources/Detail.aspx?topic=2010_Food_Health_Survey_Consumer_Attitudes_Toward_Food_Safety_Nutrition_Health.

2. Nutritiondata.com. 2011. *Self Nutrition Data*. Accessed August 14, 2011. nutritiondata.self.com.

3. World Health Organization. 2007. *Protein and Amino Acid Requirements in Human Nutrition*. WHO Technical Report Series 935. Geneva, Switzerland: World Health Organization.

4. Millward, D. Joe. 2004. "Macronutrient intakes as determinants of dietary protein and amino acid adequacy." *Journal of Nutrition* 134(6 suppl):1588S–1596S.

5. Vegan Outreach. 2010. "Protein." Accessed July 18, 2011. veganhealth.org/articles/protein.

6. Venderley, Angela M., and Wayne W. Campbell. 2006. "Vegetarian diets: Nutritional considerations for athletes." *Sports Medicine* 36(4):293–305.

7. Nieman, David C. 1999. "Physical fitness and vegetarian diets: Is there a relation?" *American Journal of Clinical Nutrition* 70(3 suppl):570S–575S.

8. Craig, Winston J., Ann Reed Mangels, and American Dietetic Association. 2009. "Position of the American Dietetic Association: Vegetarian diets." *Journal of the American Dietetic Association* 109(7):1266–1282.

9. Young, Vernon R., and Peter L. Pellett. 1994. "Plant proteins in relation to human protein and amino acid nutrition." *American Journal of Clinical Nutrition* 59 (5 suppl): 1203S–1212S.

10. Millward, D. Joe. 1999. "The nutritional value of plant-based diets in relation to human amino acid and protein requirements." *Proceedings of the Nutrition Society* 58(2):249–260.

11. Tome, Daniel, and Cecile Bos. 2007. "Lysine requirement through the human life cycle." *Journal of Nutrition* 137(6):1642S–1645S.

12. Millward, D. Joe, and Alan A. Jackson. 2004. "Protein/energy ratios of current diets in developed and developing countries compared with a safe protein/energy ratio: Implications for recommended protein and amino acid intakes." *Public Health Nutrition* 7(3):387–405.

13. Humane Society of the United States. "An HSUS report: The welfare of animals in the meat, egg, and dairy industries." Accessed August 28, 2010. humanesociety.org/assets/pdfs/farm/welfare_overview.pdf.

Chapter 8

1. Malik, Vasanti S., Matthias B. Schulze, and Frank B. Hu. 2006. "Intake of sugar-sweetened beverages and weight gain: A systematic review." *American Journal of Clinical Nutrition* 84(2):274–288.

2. Yang, Qing. 2010. "Gain weight by 'going diet'? Artificial sweeteners and the neurobiology of sugar cravings." *Yale Journal of Biology and Medicine* 83(2):101–108.

3. Mattes, Richard D., and Barry M. Popkin. 2009. "Nonnutritive sweetener consumption in humans: Effects on appetite and food intake and their putative mechanisms." *American Journal of Clinical Nutrition* 89(1):1–14.

4. Nettleton, Jennifer A., et al. 2009. "Diet soda intake and risk of incident metabolic syndrome and type 2 diabetes in the Multi-Ethnic Study of Atherosclerosis (MESA)." *Diabetes Care* 32(4):688–694.

5. Ferreira, Maria Pontes, and M. K. Suzy Weems. 2008. "Alcohol consumption by aging adults in the United States: Health benefits and detriments." *Journal of the American Dietetic Association* 108(10):1668–1676.

6. Ferreira, Maria Pontes, and Darryn Willoughby. 2008. "Alcohol consumption: The good, the bad, and the indifferent." *Applied Physiology, Nutrition, and Metabolism* 33(1):12–20.

7. Suter, Paolo M., and Angelo Tremblay. 2005. "Is alcohol a risk factor for weight gain and obesity?" *Critical Reviews in Clinical Laboratory Sciences* 42(3):197–227.

Chapter 9

1. New World Encyclopedia contributors. 2008. "McDonalds." *New World Encyclopedia*. Accessed August 23, 2010. newworldencyclopedia.org/entry/McDonalds.

2. U.S. Department of Agriculture Economic Research Service. 2008. "Food CPI and expenditures: Table 7." Accessed August 23, 2010. ers.usda.gov/Briefing/CPIFoodAndExpenditures/Data/Expenditures_tables/table7.htm.

3. Stein, Jeannine. 2010. "Americans may be running up the calorie count when dining out." *Los Angeles Times*, February 22. Accessed August 23, 2010. articles.latimes.com/2010/feb/22/health/la-he-0222-restaurant-details-20100222.

4. Rydell, Sarah A., et al. 2008. "Why eat at fast-food restaurants: Reported reasons among frequent consumers." *Journal of the American Dietetic Association* 108(12):2066–2070.

5. American Academy of Pediatrics, Committee on Communications. 2006. "Children, adolescents, and advertising." *Pediatrics* 118(6):2563–2569.

6. Consumers Union. 2005. "New report shows food industry advertising overwhelms government's '5 A Day' campaign to fight obesity and promote healthy eating." Accessed August 23, 2010. consumersunion.org/pub/core_health_care/002657.html.

7. McNally, Alex. 2008. "Industry is taking healthy eating seriously, poll finds." *Food Navigator USA*. Accessed August 23, 2010. www.foodnavigator-usa.com/Science/Industry-is-taking-healthy-eating-seriously-poll-finds.

8. Levitt, Steven D., and Stephen J. Dubner. 2005. *Freakonomics: A Rogue Economist Explores the Hidden Side of Everything*, page 328. New York: William Morrow.

9. Kechagias, Stergios, et al. 2008. "Fast-food-based hyper-alimentation can induce rapid and profound elevation of serum alanine aminotransferase in healthy subjects." *Gut* 57(5):649–654.

10. Vogel, Robert A., Mary C. Corretti, and Gary D. Plotnick. 1997. "Effect of a single high-fat meal on endothelial function in healthy subjects." *American Journal of Cardiology* 79(3):350–354.

Chapter 10

1. U.S. Department of Labor Bureau of Labor Statistics. 2009. "Economic News Release: Table 8. Time spent in primary activities . . . ." Accessed August 24, 2010. bls.gov/news.release/atus.t08.htm.

2. University of California. 2004. "Americans spend more energy watching TV than on exercise." *UC Newsroom*. Accessed August 24, 2010. universityofcalifornia.edu/news/article/6189.

3. Weber, Christopher L., and H. Scott Matthews. 2008. "Food-miles and the relative climate impacts of food choices in the United States." *Environmental Science and Technology* 42(10):3508–3513.

4. McWilliams, James E. 2009. *Just Food: Where Locavores Get It Wrong and How We Can Truly Eat Responsibly*, page 126. New York: Little, Brown, and Company

Chapter 11

1. Jakicic, John M., et al. 2008. "Effect of exercise on 24-month weight loss maintenance in overweight women." *Archives of Internal Medicine* 168(14):1550–1559.

2. Slentz, Cris A., et al. 2004. "Effects of the amount of exercise on body weight, body composition, and measures of central obesity: STRRIDE: A randomized controlled study." *Archives of Internal Medicine* 164(1):31–39.

3. Jakicic, John M., et al. 2003. "Effect of exercise duration and intensity on weight loss in overweight, sedentary women: A randomized trial." *Journal of the American Medical Association* 290(10):1323–1330.

4. Ruiz, Jonatan R., et al. 2006. "Relations of total physical activity and intensity to fitness and fatness in children: The European Youth Heart Study." *American Journal of Clinical Nutrition* 84(2):299–303.

5. Waters, Debra L., et al. 2010. "Advantages of dietary, exercise-related, and therapeutic interventions to prevent and treat sarcopenia in adults patients: An update." *Clinical Interventions in Aging* 2010(5):259–270.

6. Yoshioka, Mayumi, et al. 2001. "Impact of high-intensity exercise on energy expenditure, lipid oxidation, and body fatness." *International Journal of Obesity and Related Metabolic Disorders* 25(3):332–339.

7. Tremblay, Angelo, et al. 1990. "Effect of intensity of physical activity on body fatness and fat distribution." *American Journal of Clinical Nutrition* 51(2):153–157.

8. Tremblay, Angelo, Jean-Aime Simoneau, and Claude Bouchard. 1994. "Impact of exercise intensity on body fatness and skeletal muscle metabolism." *Metabolism* 43(7):814–818.

9. Amati, Francesca, et al. 2008. "Separate and combined effects of exercise training and weight loss on exercise efficiency and substrate oxidation." *Journal of Applied Physiology* 105(3):825–831.

Chapter 12

1. Bassett, David R., Patrick L. Schneider, and Gertrude E. Huntington. 2004. "Physical activity in an Old Order Amish community." *Medicine and Science in Sports and Exercise* 36(1):79–85.

Chapter 13

1. National Sleep Foundation Official Website. 2010. "Sleep in America Poll." Accessed March 8, 2010. sleepfoundation.org/article/sleep-america-polls/2010-sleep-and-ethnicity.

2. Gangwisch, James E., et al. 2005. "Inadequate sleep as a risk factor for obesity: Analyses of the NHANES I." *Sleep* 28(10):1289–1296.

3. Prinz, Patricia. 2004. "Sleep, appetite, and obesity—What is the link?" *PLoS Medicine* 1(3):e61.

4. Gillian, J. Christian. 2002. "How long can humans stay awake?" *Scientific American*, March 25. Accessed August 25, 2010. scientificamerican.com/article.cfm?id=how-long-can-humans-stay.

5. Dawson, Drew, and Kathryn Reid. 1997. "Fatigue, alcohol, and performance impairment." *Nature* 388(6639):235.

6. Arnedt, J. Todd, et al. 2001. "How do prolonged wakefulness and alcohol compare in the decrements they produce on a simulated driving task?" *Accident: Analysis and Prevention* 33(3):337–344.

7. Flier, Jeffrey S., and Joel K. Elmquist. 2004. "A good night's sleep: Future antidote to the obesity epidemic?" *Annals of Internal Medicine* 141(11):885–886.

8. Spiegel, Karine, Rachel Leproult, and Eve Van Cauter. 1999. "Impact of sleep debt on metabolic and endocrine function." *Lancet* 354(9188):1435–1439.

9. Spiegel, Karine, et al. 2004. "Sleep curtailment in healthy young men is associated with decreased leptin levels, elevated ghrelin levels, and increased hunger and appetite." *Annals of Internal Medicine* 141(11):846–850.

10. Spiegel, Karine, et al. 2005. "Sleep loss: A novel risk factor for insulin resistance and type 2 diabetes." *Journal of Applied Physiology* 99(5):2008–2019.

11. Sekine, Michikazu, et al. 2002. "A dose-response relationship between short sleeping hours and childhood obesity: Results of the Toyama Birth Cohort Study." *Child: Care, Health, and Development* 28(2):163–170.

12. Dzaja, Andrea, et al. 2004. "Sleep enhances nocturnal plasma ghrelin levels in healthy subjects." *American Journal of Physiology: Endocrinology and Metabolism* 286(6):e963–e967.

Chapter 14

1. Liu, Yijun, et al. 2010. "Food addiction and obesity: Evidence from bench to bedside." *Journal of Psychoactive Drugs* 42(2):133–145.

2. Pecina, Susana, and Kyle S. Smith. 2010. "Hedonic and motivational roles of opioids in food reward: Implications for overeating disorders." *Pharmacology, Biochemistry, and Behavior* 97(1):34–46.

3. Moran, Victoria. 2009. "Self-esteem, self-worth, and self-love, part 2." *Your Charmed Life* (blog). *Beliefnet.* Accessed August 14, 2011. blog.beliefnet.com/yourcharmedlife/2009/04/self-esteem-self-worth-and-self-love-part-2.html.

4. Zadoff, Allen. 2007. *Hungry: Lessons Learned on the Journey from Fat to Thin*, pages 77–78. New York: De Capo Press.

5. Centers for Disease Control and Prevention. 2011. "Alcohol and Public Health." Accessed August 14, 2011. cdc.gov/alcohol.

Chapter 15

1. Johnson, Nicholas, quoted in *Twenty Questions about Youth and the Media*, edited by Sharon R. Mazzarella, page 69. New York: Peter Lang Publishing.

2. Batada, Ameena, et al. 2008. "Nine out of 10 food advertisements shown during Saturday morning children's television programming are for foods high in fat, sodium, or added sugars, or low in nutrients." *Journal of the American Dietetic Association* 108(4):673–678.

3. Taveras, Elsie M., et al. 2010. "Racial/ethnic differences in early-life risk factors for childhood obesity." *Pediatrics* 125(4):686–695.

4. Christakis, Nicholas A., and James H. Fowler. 2009. *Connected: The Surprising Power of Our Social Networks and How They Shape Our Lives.* Boston: Little, Brown, and Company.

5. Christakis, Nicholas A., and James H. Fowler. 2007. "The spread of obesity in a large social network over 32 years." *New England Journal of Medicine* 357(4):370–379.

Chapter 16

1. Ernersson, Asa, Fredrik H. Nystrom, and Torbjorn Lindstrom. 2010. "Long-term increase of fat mass after a four week intervention with fast food based hyper-alimentation and limitation of physical activity." *Nutrition and Metabolism* (London) 7(1):68.

Chapter 17

1. Burke, Lora E., et al. 2008. "A descriptive study of past experiences with weight-loss treatment." *Journal of the American Dietetic Association* 108(4):640–647.

2. Nielsen. 2010. "A2/M2 Three Screen Report." Accessed August 23, 2010. kr.en.nielsen.com/site/documents/A2M23ScreensFINAL1Q09.pdf.

3. Singh, Sonal, Yoon K. Loke, and Curt D. Furberg. 2007. "Long-term risk of cardiovascular events with rosiglitazone: A meta-analysis." *Journal of the American Medical Association* 298(10):1189–1195.

4. Stagnitti, Marie N. 2008. "Trends in statins utilization and expenditures for the U.S. civilian noninstitutionalized population, 2000 and 2005." Medical Expenditure Panel Survey Statistical Brief 205. Rockville, MD: Agency for Healthcare Research and Quality.

5. Loke, Yoon K., Amal N. Trivedi, and Sonal Singh. 2008. "Meta-analysis: Gastrointestinal bleeding due to interaction between selective serotonin uptake inhibitors and non-steroidal anti-inflammatory drugs." *Alimentary Pharmacology and Therapeutics* 27(1):31–40.

6. U.S. Food and Drug Administration. 2009. "Meridia (sibutramine hydrochloride): Early communication about an ongoing safety review." Accessed August 28, 2010. fda.gov/Safety/MedWatch/SafetyInformation/SafetyAlertsforHumanMedicalProducts/ucm191655.htm.

7. Associated Press. 2009. "FDA probes weight-loss pill Alli over liver damage reports." *USA Today*. Accessed August 28, 2010. usatoday.com/news/health/weightloss/2009-08-24-alli-liver_N.htm.

8. Perrone, Matthew. 2008. "FDA reports deaths with diabetes drug Byetta." *Fox News*, August 18. Accessed August 28, 2010. foxnews.com/wires/2008Aug18/0,4670,DiabetesDrugFDAWarning,00.html.

9. Robbins, John. 2011. *The Food Revolution: How Your Diet Can Help Save Your Life and Our World*, page 25. San Francisco: Conari Press.

Chapter 20

1. Krzyzewski, Mike. 2000. *Leading with the Heart: Coach K's Successful Strategies for Basketball*, page 3. New York: Hachette Book Group.

Index

Page references in *italics* refer to illustrations or sidebars.

C

G

M

N

R

S

T

U

V

W

Y

Z

About the Author

Ryan Andrews completed his education and training in exercise physiology, nutrition, and dietetics at the University of Northern Colorado, Kent State University, and Johns Hopkins Medicine. He is a dietitian and strength and conditioning specialist and works with various nonprofit organizations. Ryan has given numerous presentations and written hundreds of articles about nutrition, exercise, and health. He currently serves as a coach with Precision Nutrition, offering life changing, research-driven, nutrition coaching for everyone (precisionnutrition.com).